THE ESSENTIALS OF VETERINARY POINT OF CARE ULTRASOUND

Pleural Space and Lung

Plaza Antonio Beltrán Martínez n.° 1, planta 8 - letra I
(Centro empresarial El Trovador)
50002 Zaragoza - Spain

First printing: January 2022

Illustrator:
Jacob Gragera Artal

ISBN: 978-84-18020-50-6
DL: Z 1758-2021

Design, layout and printing:
Grupo Asís Biomedia, SL
www.grupoasis.com
info@grupoasis.com

edra is an imprint of Grupo Asís

VIDEOS INCLUDED

THE ESSENTIALS OF VETERINARY POINT OF CARE ULTRASOUND

Pleural Space and Lung

Søren Boysen
Kris Gommeren
Serge Chalhoub

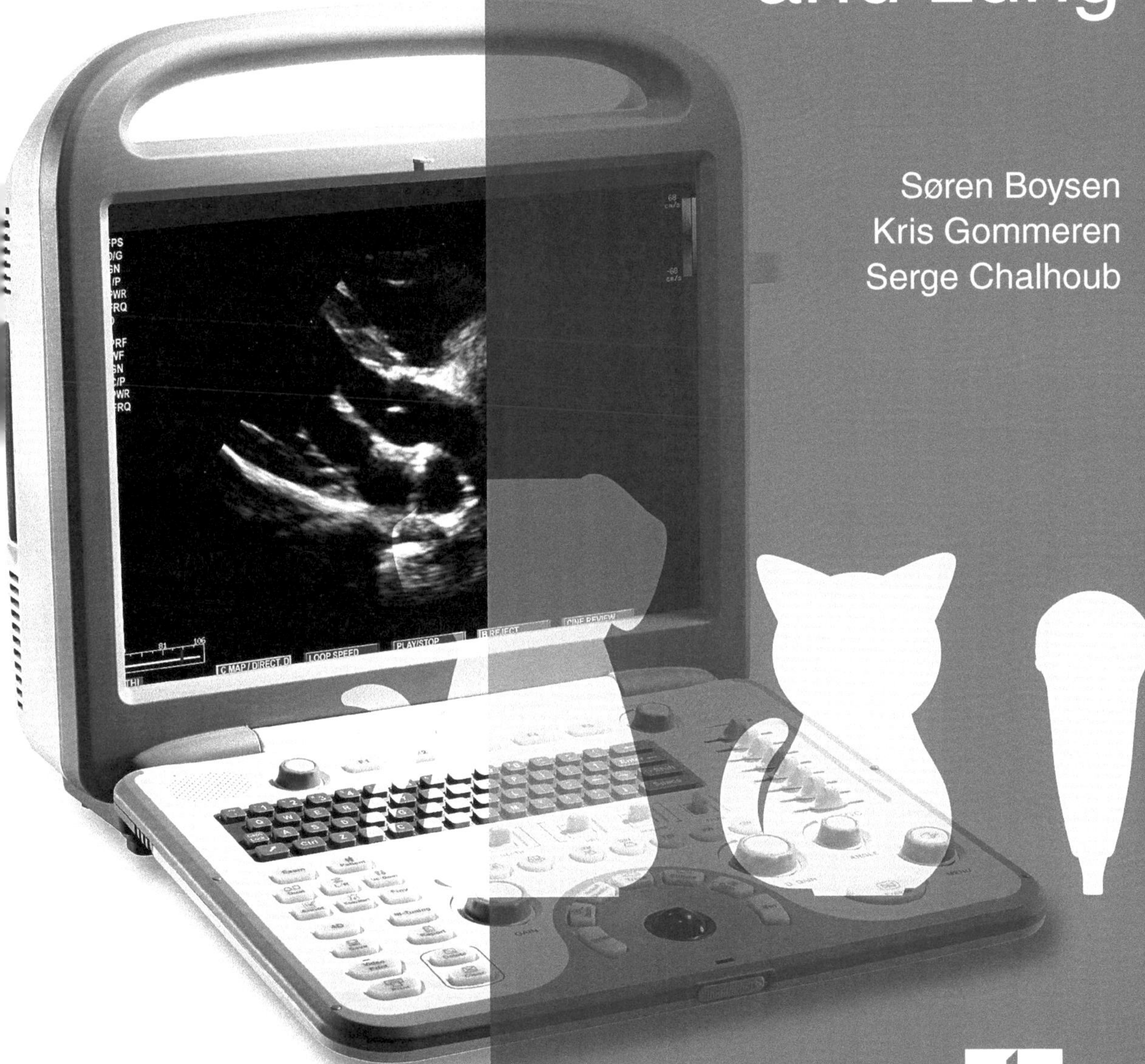

edra

THE AUTHORS

Søren Boysen

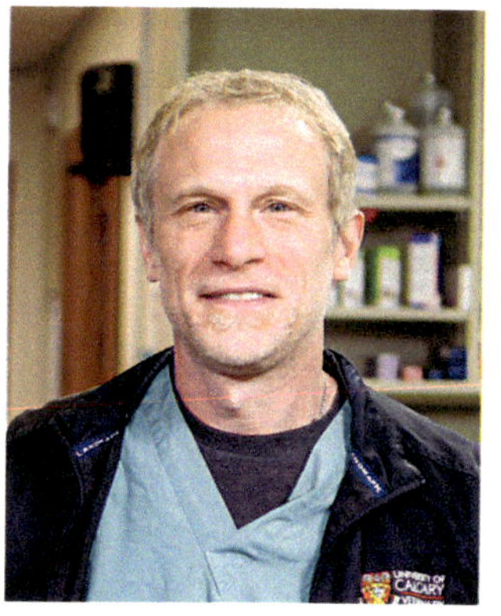

Dr. Søren Boysen obtained his DVM from the University of Saskatchewan (Canada), completed a small animal internship at the Atlantic Veterinary College (Canada), and a residency at Tufts University (United States), becoming a diplomate of the American College of Veterinary Emergency and Critical Care in 2003. He is the former Chief of Small Animal Emergency and Critical Care at the University of Montreal, and currently a full professor of veterinary emergency and critical care at the University of Calgary. Extensively published, and a recipient of numerous teaching and research excellence awards, he has become an internationally recognized speaker. Although he loves all things emergency and critical care, he is considered a pioneer of veterinary point-of-care ultrasound (POCUS), having published the first small animal Focused Assessment of Sonography for Trauma (FAST) exam in collaboration with colleagues from Tufts. With many great colleagues from around the world he continues to actively research and develop ultrasound training techniques, education programs, and workshops for nonspecialist practitioners. Along with point-of-care ultrasound, his research interests include hemorrhage, coagulation, and perfusion.

Kris Gommeren

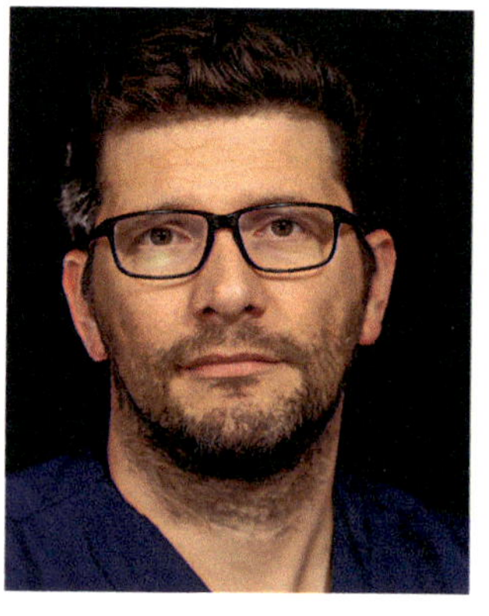

Kris Gommeren graduated in 2002 from Ghent University, where he subsequently performed an internship and a residency in internal medicine, becoming a Diplomate of the European College of Veterinary Internal Medicine in 2009. After his residency he briefly worked in a private referral practice, but soon moved to the University of Liège, where he has been in charge of the Emergency and Critical Care Service since 2008. He completed a PhD on the effects of systemic inflammation on the cardiovascular system. In 2017 he became a Diplomate of the European College of Veterinary Emergency and Critical Care. Kris has been actively involved in the European Veterinary Emergency and Critical Care Society (EVECCS) for over ten years. His main fields of interest are point-of-care ultrasound, the cardiovascular system, fluid therapy including the assessment of volume status, as well as transfusion medicine.

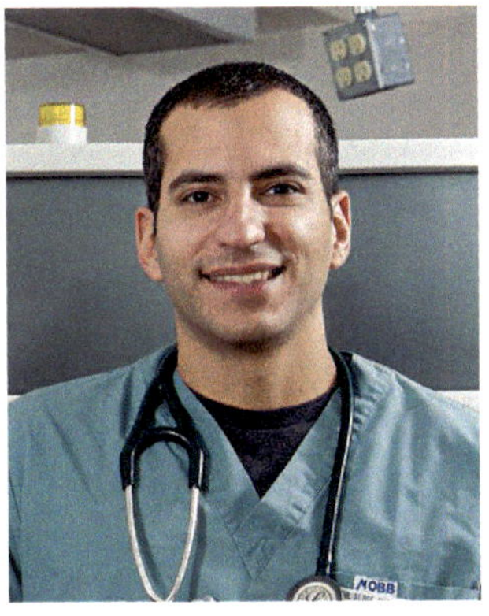

Serge Chalhoub

Born and raised in Montreal, Dr. Chalhoub graduated from the DVM program at the Faculty of Veterinary Medicine (FMV) of the University of Montreal in 2004. He then completed a one-year rotating small animal internship at the same institution. After working for two years as a general practitioner and emergency veterinarian at the DMV Centre in Montreal, Dr. Chalhoub pursued a residency in small animal internal medicine at the Animal Medical Center (AMC) in New York City. Once completed in 2009 he stayed on at the AMC as their first renal/hemodialysis fellow. During this time, he was also trained in interventional radiology/endoscopy. Dr. Chalhoub is currently a senior instructor at the University of Calgary's Faculty of Veterinary Medicine (UCVM). He was the recipient of the 2013 Canadian Veterinary Medical Association's Teacher of the Year Award, the 2015 University of Calgary Team Teacher of the Year Award, and the 2017 Carl J. Norden Distinguished Teacher Award. He is the coordinator of the UCVM-CUPS Pet Health Clinic for disadvantaged Calgarians. He has authored and coauthored numerous scientific articles and book chapters on veterinary point-of-care ultrasound, renal and urinary medicine.

FOREWORD

Almost two decades have passed since Søren Boysen published on the use of ultrasound in the emergency room. In that time a lot has changed in the use of point of care ultrasound (POCUS). The increasing affordability and portability of ultrasound machines alongside a greater understanding of the use of ultrasound in veterinary emergency and critical care (ECC), not only from extrapolating from our human medicine colleagues, but also our own research, has meant that ECC veterinarians can use POCUS for increased benefit for their patients, in a reliable, efficient, and safe way.

With any new application of a diagnostic imaging tool, it is important to consider what is a normal image, what is abnormal image and what do the results mean in the clinical context? It is paramount to interpret the images alongside the clinical history and physical examination to minimise diagnostic error. This is the core of the book; from the POCUS techniques recommended, to the interpretation of the images the authors emphasise how POCUS can help answer key clinical questions in ECC patients.

The authors, Søren Boysen, Kris Gommeren and Serge Chalboub have been long term collaborators in the POCUS space, as well as being lead researchers in the area they also dedicate a large amount of their spare time to teaching POCUS through articles, practical courses and delivering lectures at national and international conferences. Their upbeat personalities and relaxed styles are infectious, as is their passion for POCUS, which comes across in abundance with their latest endeavour; this book.

They have created an extremely practical book packed with high quality diagrams, images and flow charts. The standardised binary question approach used throughout the book allows for real time practical application of POCUS. The inclusion of key points section alongside common pitfalls are appreciated additions for the busy clinician. It is packed with QR codes which allows for easy access to videos of everything that you could possibly want to see.

This book is a must have for those that use POCUS in any capacity, as a reference, refresher, and reminder; we could not endorse it more.

Dominic Barfield & Laura Cole

Dominic Barfield: President of the European College of Veterinary Emergency and Critical Care

Laura Cole: Vice-President of the Veterinary Emergency and Critical Care Ultrasound Society

PREFACE

This book titled *Essentials of Veterinary Point-of-Care Ultrasound. Pleural Space and Lung* is designed to be a reference for both the new and experienced veterinary point-of-care sonographer. It includes many key tips, tricks and any additional information that we as nonradiologists or cardiologists have found helpful in assessing the pleural space and lung. It covers a step-by-step how-to approach to performing pleural space and lung ultrasound and uses a binary question approach to allow novices and experts alike to master and grow their skills. Relevant sonographic anatomy of the pleural space and lung as well as general techniques are reviewed. Consideration of how patient positioning impacts localization of pathology such as fluid and air, and how to modify protocols to increase the chances of detecting pathology based on patient position are presented. The importance of creating PLUS profiles by mapping multiple regions of the lung and pleural space for the presence or absence of pathology, in conjunction with other POCUS, history, clinical and diagnostic findings is emphasized. Finally, the book provides specific techniques, key criteria to assess, and image interpretation for each of the following binary questions regarding the pleural space and lung: "Is there pneumothorax?", "Is there pleural effusion?", "Are there increased B lines?" "Is there lung consolidation?", "Is there pleural thickening?", and "Are there pleural irregularities?". What each of these findings represent and how to differentiate them from other pathologies is discussed. Finally, limitations and pitfalls for each binary question are also covered. This book should be helpful for any veterinarian, vet student, intern, resident or even technician who is currently learning or practicing veterinary point-of-care ultrasound.

The authors

TABLE OF CONTENTS

01

INTRODUCTION

EVOLUTION OF PLEURA AND LUNG ULTRASOUND (PLUS)

Thoracic veterinary point-of-care ultrasound (POCUS) has evolved greatly over the last several years as its application into clinical veterinary medicine has grown. In 2008, Lisciandro et al. published a veterinary thoracic focused assessment with sonography for trauma (TFAST) protocol to evaluate thoracic injury in dogs predominantly placed in right lateral recumbency using two bilateral sonographic windows: the chest tube site and the pericardial site[1]. The initial objective was to identify trauma-induced thoracic injury, particularly pneumothorax via assessment of lung sliding (glide sign) at the chest tube site, and pleural and pericardial effusion, at the pericardial site. Following the 4-point exam, a 5-point TFAST protocol, which included the subxiphoid site, demonstrated that thoracic POCUS is not limited to the trauma setting and may be beneficial in the triage assessment of all unstable animals[2]. However, given TFAST was not originally designed to assess more than a single sonographic window of lung surface on either hemithorax (e.g. it only assessed a single intercostal space at the chest tube site), numerous veterinary lung ultrasound protocols were quickly developed to assess multiple lung regions for the presence of lung pathology[3-7]. Most recently, newer thoracic veterinary POCUS approaches that incorporate pleura, pleural space and lung under the same umbrella have been developed[6,7].

Unfortunately, the accuracy of thoracic POCUS to identify pleural space pathology in dogs and cats has been met with conflicting results[8,9]. The original TFAST study demonstrated there is a steep learning curve to diagnose pneumothorax in dogs with an overall sensitivity of 45 % for less experienced sonographers, which increases up to 95 % when performed by experts, although the true sensitivity is unknown as TFAST was not compared to the reference standard computed tomography (CT)[1]. The accuracy of TFAST to identify other pleural space pathology, lung pathology, and pericardial effusion was not reported in the original study, likely due to the low incidence of these pathologies being identified and lack of a reference standard for comparison[1]. Computed tomography is the reference standard for detecting lung and pleural space lesions such as small quantities of pleural effusion or air, which may not be related to clinical signs and may not be detectable with TFAST[8,9]. Subsequent veterinary studies in dogs and cats showed only poor to fair accuracy of TFAST and veterinary bedside lung ultrasound evaluation (Vet BLUE) compared to CT for the diagnosis of pneumothorax and pleural effusion, respectively, although results should be interpreted with caution as the methodology used varied slightly between studies and only small case numbers were included[8,9].

The conflicting results between early thoracic POCUS protocols and CT for detection of pleural space pathology are probably multifactorial, and likely depends on the experience of the sonographer, underlying pathologies, patient positioning, scanning protocol, and criteria used to diagnose these pathologies[6,8,9]. Some authors also suggest TFAST and Vet BLUE sites are not the most sensitive locations to detect smaller volume pneumothoraces and pleural effusions[8,9]. Two recent studies support this hypothesis, demonstrating a higher probability of detecting small volume pleural effusion in sternal/standing dogs when the transducer is orientated parallel to the ribs and more ventral regions of the pleural space are evaluated compared to the pericardial site[6,10]. Furthermore, TFAST and some lung ultrasound scanning techniques evaluate fixed external anatomic landmarks (i.e. ribs spaces) while ignoring the considerable variation of sonographically-defined thoracic borders (e.g. due to breed differences, patient size, fat content, respiratory effort, etc.) and how patient positioning affects the location of certain pathology due to the effects of gravity. Although most dogs in the original TFAST study were positioned in right lateral recumbency, some were evaluated in left lateral and in sternal recumbency, but the same chest tube and pericardial sites were used regardless of patient position, size or breed[1]. This may have impacted results as fluid and air will accumulate in different locations depending on the position in which patients are evaluated (lateral vs. sternal or standing)[1,6]. In addition, differences have been found in relation to what clinicians include within thoracic POCUS exams, likely because protocols have changed over time. In a Pan-Canadian survey regarding the use of POCUS, thoracic ultrasound had significant variability in terms of what clinicians evaluate in their TFAST and lung ultrasound protocols[11]. The use of the term "chest tube" to describe transducer locations may further contribute to the variation noted between studies and clinicians as it lacks precision: thoracostomy tube placement sites vary in the literature and based on the reason thoracostomy tubes are placed (fluid vs. air)[12-15], leading to different TFAST sites being used by different clinicians. Thoracostomy tubes are also not traditionally placed at the most caudodorsal site of the pleural space[12-15], which is where smaller volume pneumothoraces are most likely to occur in sternal/standing patients.

In contrast to the mixed results of identifying pleural space pathology, research shows veterinary thoracic POCUS is accurate at detecting lung pathology, particularly increased B lines associated with congestive heart failure and pulmonary contusions, although its accuracy to detect other abnormal lung findings beyond increased B lines (e.g. lung consolidation) is in its infancy in veterinary medicine and only just starting to be investigated[8,16-18]. Although all veterinary lung ultrasound protocols developed to date show promise, comparison between different lung ultrasound protocols for detection of pleural space and lung pathology requires further investigation.

Due to the limitations and variable results reported above, the authors suggest a modified approach to sonographically evaluating the pleura and lung in veterinary patients: the clinical situation encountered should dictate how thoracic POCUS is applied and different protocols should be used to identify different pathologies using a specific clinically driven (often binary) question approach.

The authors recommend using sonographically-defined pleura and lung borders of the thoracic cavity versus external fixed anatomical sites, and considering patient positioning to increase the sensitivity and specificity in finding underlying pathologies. It is particularly important for novice sonographers to understand anatomic landmarks and how physiology and pathophysiology impact findings.

Thus, instead of applying a single protocol to all patients, the sonographer should ask what specific pathology needs to be ruled in or out, and how patient position affects where pathology accumulates. In other words, the clinician asks what questions need to be answered, and modifies POCUS formats to answer these questions (in contrast to a fixed protocol being rigidly applied in all cases).

In addition, sonographers should be familiar with pleura and lung borders to increase the odds of identifying specific pathologies, and to orientate the operator to where they are on the thorax, which helps avoid interpreting normal anatomic structures for pathology. This has resulted in development of the Calgary pleura and lung ultrasound (PLUS) approach.

It becomes important to standardize the approach to PLUS so that the information stays objective and translatable between clinicians.

The PLUS approach is situationally driven, and prioritizes the most pressing clinical question to be investigated if the animal is dyspneic and/or unstable; however, PLUS can also be used as an adjunct to the physical exam in any patient to advance further diagnostics and therapeutics (such as thoracocentesis), to serially monitor any change in the patient's PLUS findings (improved/worsened), and also as a daily evaluation of the patient until discharge (Fig. 1). In essence PLUS is applied similarly to the more broadly applied 5 T's of POCUS: trauma, triage, treatment, tracking, and total.

IMPORTANT CONSIDERATIONS FOR PLUS

PLUS provides clinically significant information that is otherwise unattainable on physical examination alone, and is therefore complimentary to triage, physical examination and other point of care diagnostic and clinical tests or findings: It does not replace them. Thus, it is designed to quickly narrow differential diagnoses and rapidly rule out life threatening conditions and further direct diagnostics and therapies.

Presenting complaint, triage and physical exam

As stated above, PLUS is situationally dictated and therefore applied differently depending on the clinical setting encountered (Fig. 1). Immediate clinical scenario and presenting complaint must be considered in order to prioritize the order of scanning prior to performing all components of PLUS or POCUS.

For example, if a patient presents for respiratory distress PLUS is performed before abdominal POCUS. Based on the initial presenting complaint or clinical signs/exam, various scenarios exist for the application of PLUS. If a hit-by-car patient presents with significant respiratory distress and has decreased breath sounds dorsally, in addition to the triage exam and emergency therapy including sedation, pain medications, and oxygen, the immediate PLUS exam should be focused on assessing for pneumothorax, which if present is immediately addressed. In this specific clinical scenario, the presenting complaint and initial triage exam dictates the most important clinical (often binary) question to answer first: "is there

Figure 1. Calgary PLUS approach. MEDB: minimum emergency database.

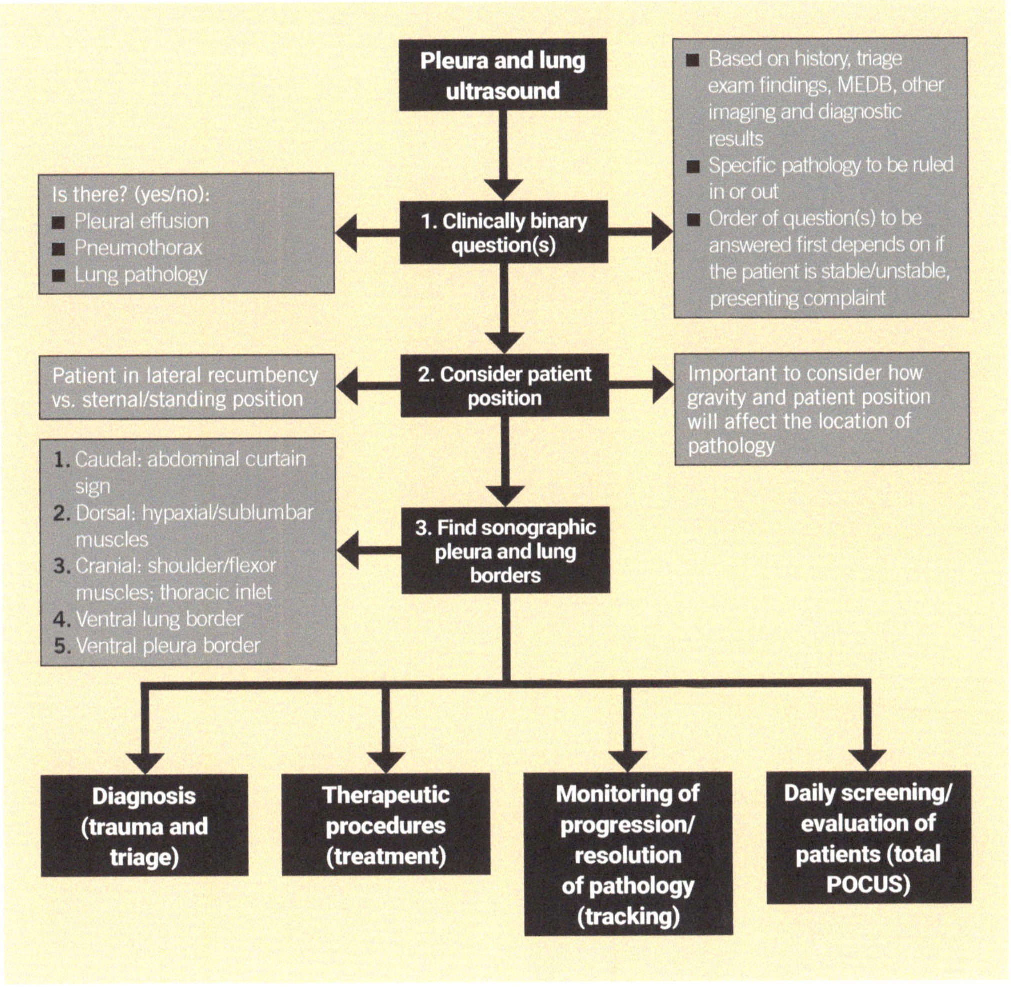

pneumothorax (yes/no)?" (see Chapter 4). A full physical exam and full PLUS or POCUS examination is not immediately recommended if the patient is unstable, and time is of the essence.

Similar to a triage exam being followed by a more comprehensive physical exam, once the patient is stable and life-threatening conditions have been dealt with, more comprehensive total POCUS evaluations (i.e. full PLUS and other abdominal and cardiovascular POCUS scans) can be completed. Furthermore, if the same patient has severe life-threatening respiratory distress, stabilization including thoracocentesis takes precedence.

Key point

It is important not to compromise patient safety or delay lifesaving interventions to complete the PLUS and/or a full POCUS evaluation.

Clinically driven binary questions

A clinically driven, often binary question approach allows the rapid and thorough investigation of prioritized specific clinically-relevant questions that will assist in further triage of the patient, especially if unstable, or in the systemic evaluation of stable patients. Not having a clinically driven question to answer can lead to "fishing expeditions" where the transducer is randomly placed on the patient in the hope of finding something without knowing what to look for or where to locate it.

A clinically driven, often binary question approach must be used to prioritize clinically-relevant questions and to keep POCUS focused and standardized.

For example, if an open-ended approach is used when a cat comes in unstable and dyspneic, the following question might be asked "why is this cat dyspneic?" This will result in multiple differential diagnoses that fail to narrow the possibilities in a timely fashion in the emergency setting. Thus, an open–ended approach is more appropriate for stable or chronically ill patients with less specific signs, and that require an extensive work-up when urgency is not a priority. If a clinically driven POCUS approach is applied based on initial triage findings and the presenting complaint, the urgent question becomes "in this unstable dyspneic cat, is pleural space or lung pathology present?", which leads to a subsequent set of binary questions; "is pleural effusion present (yes/no)? Is pneumothorax present (yes/no)? Are increased B lines present (yes/no)? Is lung consolidation present (yes/no)?" (see subsequent Chapters). These are all questions that can quickly and confidently be assessed with PLUS, helping direct further diagnostics and therapy in a more efficient manner. When the patient is stable additional clinically driven PLUS and POCUS questions are assessed to avoid missing pathology.

In many settings multiple complimentary binary questions will be rapidly and chronologically answered based on clinically driven results. For example, if a Doberman presents in respiratory distress with a heart murmur and cough, the initial binary question is "are there increased B lines present (yes/no)?", which if present, may rapidly lead to the binary cardiovascular POCUS question "is the left atrium enlarged (yes/no)?". Similar to any patient evaluation, PLUS is fluid in nature and findings should only be interpreted in light of the entire clinical picture, which may lead to additional and more comprehensive POCUS evaluations as results become available and/or patient stabilization is initiated.

Finally, the question asked, even if binary, must be thoroughly answered to ensure the correct diagnosis is reached. For example, if the objective is to rule out a small volume of pleural effusion, placing the transducer at single thoracic site (e.g. at the level of the costochondral junction over the heart) is likely to miss the effusion: a thorough evaluation of the entire ventral pleural space (between the cranial and caudal PLUS borders) with the patient in a standing or sternal position, and with the transducer orientated parallel to the ribs should be completed (see Chapter 5).

Patient position

Patient position affects where pleural space pathology will be located. Fluid falls to gravity-dependent regions and air rises to gravity-independent regions. For instance, the most sensitive location to identify a small volume of pleural effusion in a laterally recumbent patient will be at the widest gravity-dependent (lowest) site of the thorax.

However, if that same patient is in sternal recumbency, gravity will change the site pleural effusion will gravitate towards, accumulating at the most ventral regions between the lung and sternal muscles[10]. In the sternal patient, finding the ventral borders of the

Relevant binary questions

The relevant binary questions for PLUS include:

- Is there pleural effusion (yes/no)?
- Is there pneumothorax (yes/no)?
- Are there abnormal lung ultrasound findings; increased B lines and/or lung consolidations (yes/no)?
- Is there pleura thickening/irregularities and/or small subpleural consolidation (yes/no)?

Key points of the binary approach

There are several key points to consider when using a binary approach:

- The "fishing expedition", often associated with low pre-test probabilities which may lead to significant increases in the likelihood of false positive and false negative results, can be avoided by clearly defining the objectives of sonographic clinically driven binary questions.
- The binary question to answer must be kept in mind, and therefore, the order of POCUS will vary based on the clinical setting encountered. In other words, if a patient presents with dyspnea, thoracic POCUS is completed first, followed by other POCUS exams that may be applied during or following initial stabilization as dictated by the clinical situation. Within PLUS, if a patient is markedly dyspneic with decreased breath sounds ventrally, pleural effusion should be ruled out, and if present, the patient stabilized with thoracocentesis prior to completing the entire PLUS scan.
- A complete thorough sonographic assessment must be done in order to answer the specific clinically driven binary question being asked. For example, if trying to answer "are there abnormal lung ultrasound findings present?" then both sides of the thorax should be examined systematically over multiple lung regions and the PLUS profile considered (see Chapter 7).

pleura will assist in the detection of smaller volume effusion as this becomes the lowest gravity-dependent site of the thorax (Fig. 2).

Therefore, before scanning a patient, it is important to know the clinically driven question to answer, the specific pathology to look for, and to consider how the patient position will affect where to look for specific pathology. This will be further described in subsequent Chapters.

Patient position must be evaluated as this will affect where specific pathology will be located because of gravity.

Sonographically-defined pleura and lung borders

Defining sonographic pleura and lung borders and not relying on external anatomical landmarks may increase the sensitivity and

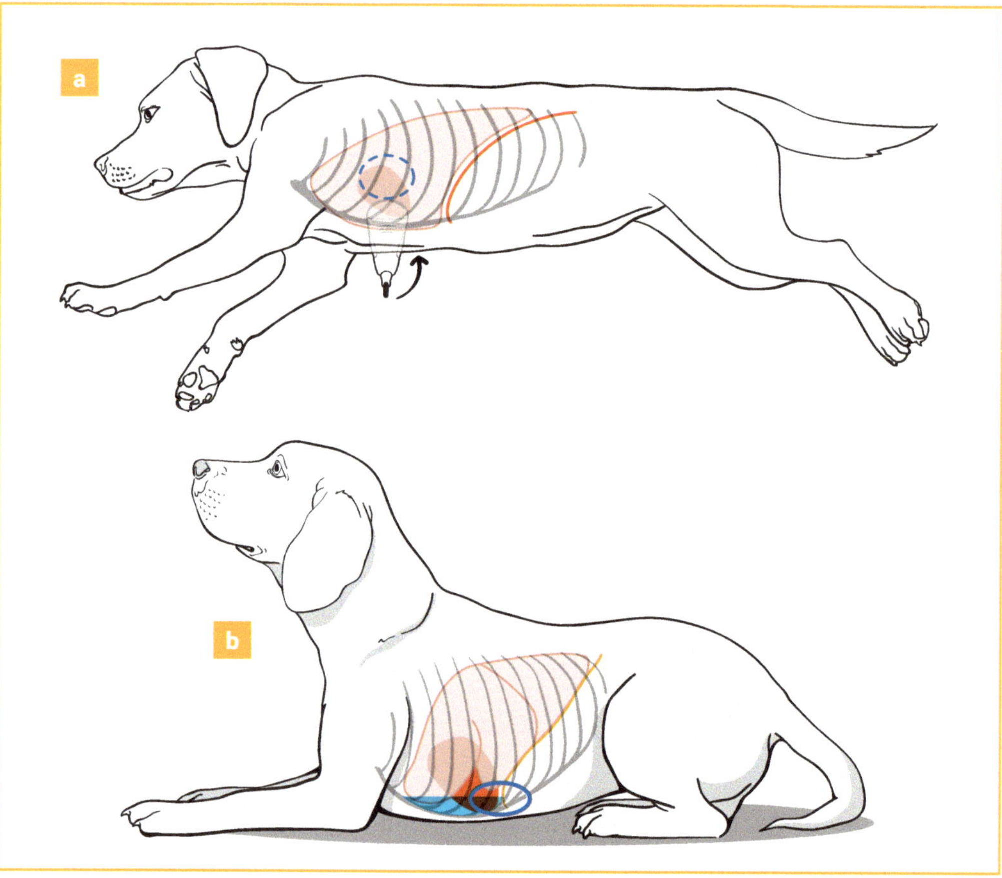

Figure 2. Patient position affects where pathology is located and the most sensitive region to detect this pathology. Patient in lateral recumbency showing small amounts of pleural effusion at the lowest gravity dependent region (blue dotted circle) of the thorax (a). Sternal or standing patient showing pleural effusion at the lowest portion of the thorax at the pericardiodiaphragmatic (blue circle) and ventral sternal regions (blue fluid) (b).

specificity of detecting pathology[6,10] and ensures that the pleura and lung, and not abdomen for instance, are being evaluated. The importance of this is highlighted by the fact that patients are not uniform in size or conformation, have varying fat content, and different underlying pathology which change defined scannable lung regions and pleura borders.

Therefore, as opposed to relying on external anatomic landmarks to estimate pleura and lung borders which vary from species to species and between individual animals, identifiable sonographically-defined pleura and lung borders should be used. There are five sonographically-defined pleura and lung borders that can be identified in healthy animals (Fig. 3):

1. The caudal border defined by the abdominal curtain sign (see Chapter 3).
2. The dorsal border defined by the hypaxial/sublumbar muscles.
3. The cranial border defined by the flexor muscles of the shoulder dorsally and the thoracic inlet ventrally (with the limb extended cranially).
4. The ventral pleura border defined by the pectoral/sternal muscles interfacing with either the lung (cranially and caudally) or heart (centrally) due to the presence of the cardiac notch.
5. The ventral lung border defined by the ventral lung margins which deviate dorsally from the ventral pleura border because of the cardiac notch.

Sonographic borders are not preserved with regards to external anatomic landmarks and will vary for each individual patient.

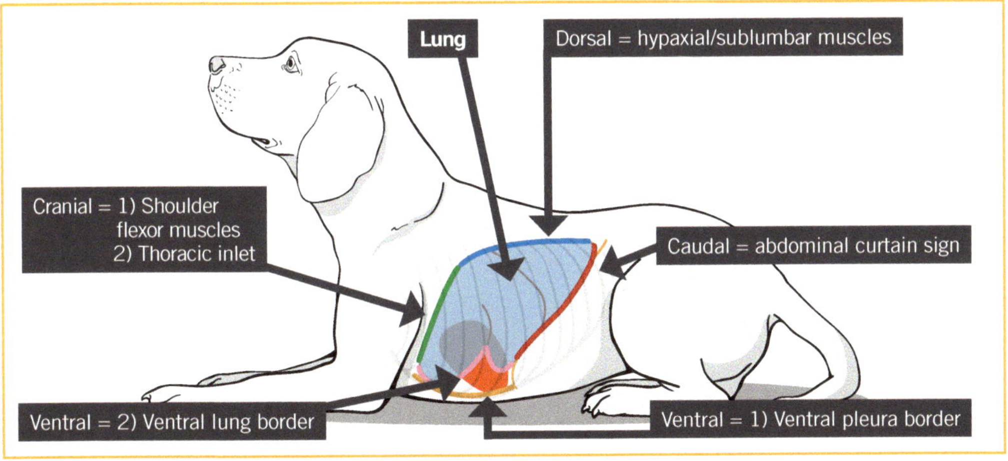

Figure 3. The five sonographically-defined pleura and lung borders of healthy patients. The caudal border is the abdominal curtain sign (red outline). The dorsal border is comprised of the hypaxial/sublumbar muscles (blue outline). The cranial border is defined by what is sonographically visible due to the musculature and presence of the thoracic limb (green outline). The ventral pleura border (orange outline) is comprised of the sternal/pectoral muscles. The ventral lung border is shown in pink.

Lung is easily defined lying between the identifiable borders. The identification of these boundaries, knowing which boundaries are most likely to result in specific pathology, and considering patient position will allow for more accurate detection of pathology regardless of breed or species. Further description of these boundaries and how to locate them will be highlighted in subsequent chapters.

SUMMARY

Pleura and lung ultrasound has evolved greatly over the last few years. The original thoracic FAST protocols primarily assessed pleural space and pericardial disease at focal external anatomic sites. More recent protocols have shown that other pathologies such as increased B lines, lung consolidation, thickened/irregular pleura and subpleural consolidations can also be detected. Evidence suggests some thoracic POCUS protocols are not accurate at detecting all underlying pleura and lung pathology. Sensitivity and reliability of thoracic POCUS may be improved by using a clinically driven (often binary) question approach, considering how patient positioning affects where pathology is most likely to accumulate, and by sonographically defining pleura and lung borders. A clinically-oriented, binary question approach allows the clinician to apply PLUS to answer important questions in an efficient prioritized but thorough manner, thereby assisting with further diagnostic and therapeutic interventions in the unstable patient. In more stable or hospitalized patients, a more comprehensive set of clinically driven binary questions should be asked and answered when there is no immediate life-threatening problem that needs to be addressed. To help with teaching, application and understanding of pleura, pleural space and lung ultrasound the authors have developed the Calgary PLUS approach.

REFERENCES

1. Lisciandro GR, Lagutchik MS, Mann KA, et al. Evaluation of a thoracic focused assessment with sonography for trauma (TFAST) protocol to detect pneumothorax and concurrent thoracic injury in 145 traumatized dogs. *J Vet Emerg Crit Care*. (2008), 18:258.
2. McMurray J, Boysen S, Chalhoub S. Focused assessment with sonography in nontraumatized dogs and cats in the emergency and critical care setting. *J Vet Emerg Crit Care (San Antonio)*. 2016, 26(1):64–73.
3. Rademacher N, Pariaut R, Pate J, et al. Transthoracic lung ultrasound in normal dogs and dogs with cardiogenic pulmonary edema: a pilot study. *Vet Radiol Ultrasound*. 2014, 55(4):447–452.
4. Vezzosi T, Mannucci T, Pistoresi A, et al. Assessment of Lung Ultrasound B-Lines in Dogs with Different Stages of Chronic Valvular Heart Disease. *J Vet Intern Med*. 2017, 31(3):700–704.
5. Lisciandro GR, Fosgate GT, Fulton RM. Frequency and number of ultrasound lung rockets (B-lines) using a regionally based lung ultrasound examination named vet BLUE (veterinary bedside lung ultrasound exam) in dogs with radiographically normal lung findings. *Vet Radiol Ultrasound*. 2014, 55(3):315–322.
6. Boysen S, McMurray J, Gommeren K. Abnormal Curtain Signs Identified With a Novel Lung Ultrasound Protocol in Six Dogs With Pneumothorax. *Front Vet Sci*. 2019, 6:291
7. Armenise A, Boysen RS, Rudloff E, et al. Veterinary-focused assessment with sonography for trauma-airway, breathing, circulation, disability and exposure: a prospective observational study in 64 canine trauma patients. *J Small Anim Pract*. 2019, 60(3):173–182.
8. Cole L, Pivetta M, Humm K. Diagnostic accuracy of a lung ultrasound protocol (Vet BLUE) for detection of pleural fluid, pneumothorax and lung pathology in dogs and cats. *J Small Anim Pract*. 2021, 62(3):178–186.
9. Walters AM, O'Brien MA, Selmic LE, et al. Evaluation of the agreement between focused assessment with sonography for trauma (AFAST/TFAST) and computed tomography in dogs and cats with recent trauma. *J Vet Emerg Crit Care (San Antonio)*. 2018, 28(5):429–435.
10. S. Boysen, S. Chalhoub, A. Romero. Veterinary point-of-care ultrasound transducer orientation for detection of pleural effusion in dog cadavers by novice sonographers: a pilot study. *Ultrasound J*. 2020, 12(Suppl 1): 45.
11. Pelchat J, Chalhoub S, Boysen S. The use of veterinary point of care ultrasound by veterinarians: a nationwide Canadian survey. *Can Vet J*. 2020, 61(12):1278–1282.
12. Del Magno S, Foglia A, Golinelli L, et al. The use of small-bore wire-guided chest drains for the management of feline pyothorax: A retrospective case series. *Open Vet J*. 2021, 10(4):443–451.
13. Valtolina C, Adamantos S. Evaluation of small-bore wire-guided chest drains for management of pleural space disease. *J Small Anim Pract*. 2009, 50(6):290–297.
14. Stillion JR, Letendre JA. A clinical review of the pathophysiology, diagnosis, and treatment of pyothorax in dogs and cats. *J Vet Emerg Crit Care (San Antonio)*. 2015 Jan-Feb, 25(1):113–129.
15. Kahn SA. Thoracostomy tube placement in the dog. *Lab Anim (NY)*. 2007, 36(3):21, 24.
16. Dicker SA, Lisciandro GR, Newell SM, Johnson JA. Diagnosis of pulmonary contusions with point-of-care lung ultrasonography and thoracic radiography compared to thoracic computed tomography in dogs with motor vehicle trauma: 29 cases (2017-2018). *J Vet Emerg Crit Care (San Antonio)*. 2020, 30(6):638–646.
17. Ward JL, Lisciandro GR, Keene BW, Tou SP, DeFrancesco TC. Accuracy of point-of-care lung ultrasonography for the diagnosis of cardiogenic pulmonary edema in dogs and cats with acute dyspnea. *J Am Vet Med Assoc*. 2017, 250(6):666–675.
18. Ward JL, Lisciandro GR, Ware WA, Miles KG, Viall AK, DeFrancesco TC. Lung ultrasonography findings in dogs with various underlying causes of cough. *J Am Vet Med Assoc*. 2019, 255(5):574–583.

02

GENERAL APPROACH

THE CALGARY PLEURA AND LUNG ULTRASOUND (PLUS) APPROACH

The Calgary Pleura and Lung Ultrasound (PLUS) approach is unique because it considers how the location of pleural space and lung pathology is affected by species and breed anatomic differences, the mechanics of breathing (lung and thoracic wall recoil), the effects of gravity, and different patient positioning, and modifies the sonographic windows evaluated accordingly. There are multiple lung ultrasound protocols currently used in veterinary medicine, all of which tend to start in the caudodorsal thoracic region at specific intercostal spaces, and all of which scan multiple lung fields. Unfortunately, consistently identifying the correct starting caudodorsal region of the thorax can be a challenge, given that the location of lung borders varies by breed, species, respiratory effort, and patient positioning. In the authors' experience, starting too low or too far cranial on the chest is the most common reason for sonographers failing to identify smaller volume pneumothorax.

An advantage of the Calgary PLUS approach is that it uses sonographically identifiable landmarks (and not set intercostal spaces) to standardize transducer location and orientate the sonographer to where they are during the scanning process. This helps to avoid the pitfalls of mistaking normal structures for pathology (e.g. gas in the stomach for B lines) and ensures the most likely areas to find pathology of the pleural space are assessed (e.g. the most caudodorsal sites for pneumothorax and the most ventral sites for fluid when the patient is in sternal recumbency or standing, and the widest parts of the thorax for patients in lateral recumbency).

Another important advantage of the Calgary PLUS approach includes evaluation of the abdominal curtain sign (vertical soft tissue-to-air interface, sonographically defined caudal lung/pleura border; see Chapter 3), which aids in the diagnosis of pleural space and lung pathology, and evaluation of the pericardiodiaphragmatic window, which helps identify and differentiate pleural and pericardial effusion. Failure to assess the ventral regions of the pleural space below the costochondral junction and not turning the transducer parallel to the ribs in the ventral thoracic regions are reasons that small-volume pleural effusion is often missed. The subxiphoid site is also included in the evaluation of the lungs and pleural space.

Depending on patient history and/or physical examination findings, not all portions of the PLUS examination need to be performed at one time. The order may vary depending upon whether life-threatening pathology is suspected and the binary question the clinician is trying to answer; the entire scan can be completed following stabilization of any life-threatening conditions.

CONTRAINDICATIONS AND COMPLICATIONS

No significant contraindications or complications are associated with PLUS examinations. PLUS is a noninvasive, rapid, repeatable, point-of-care diagnostic tool that can be performed at the time of initial patient evaluation and treatment (physical examination, blood pressure, intravenous IV catheter, IV fluids,

Indications

Dyspneic patients:

- Patients with suspected pneumothorax (e.g. dyspnea with decreased breath sounds dorsally, trauma patients).
- Patients with suspected pleural effusion (e.g. dyspnea with decreased breath sounds ventrally, cats in congestive heart failure, trauma patients).
- Patients with suspected lung pathology (e.g. crackles, cough, heart murmur, trauma, etc).

Trauma patients:

- Thoracic or generalized blunt or penetrating trauma.

Unstable patients:

- Any collapsed and/or unstable patient (e.g. elevated shock index, hyperlactatemia, unexplained hypotension, tachycardia, or decreased mentation), particularly if the underlying cause is uncertain.
- Postsurgical patients not recovering as expected.
- Any hospitalized patient that is, or becomes, unstable.

Treatment:

- To assist with ultrasound-guided procedures (i.e. thoracocentesis).

Tracking:

- To monitor progression or resolution of identified pathology.

Total:

- Following transfer to a service.
- As part of ICU patient daily management.
- Pre- and postanesthesia.

Note: All patients of the ICU service at the authors' clinic have daily systemic POCUS scans performed as part of the routine patient evaluation.

sedation, analgesia, pulse oximetry (SPO_2), minimum emergency database, etc), or as part of continued daily patient monitoring.

Stabilization efforts take priority and are not interrupted for the sake of obtaining medical imaging; therefore, the machine is brought to the patient and stabilization continued during POCUS.

SERIAL EXAMINATIONS

Serial examinations are warranted to track the development of pathology over time, to document whether it is worsening or improving, and to determine if therapy is meeting its intended goals. They are also indicated to reassess patients that did not have visible pathology at presentation, particularly those that are unstable, and/or have received significant quantities of intravascular fluid. The timing of serial examinations should be based on the overall clinical assessment of the patient, as well as consideration of the suspected disease process (e.g. a patient involved in vehicular trauma will be serially scanned for the development of pleural effusion, pneumothorax, and pulmonary contusions).

If a patient's condition fails to stabilize after therapeutic efforts, or destabilizes at any point, serial PLUS examinations should be performed.

For example, a dog that presents for vomiting, has unremarkable POCUS findings at presentation, and becomes acutely dyspneic while hospitalized on intravenous fluids, should have serial PLUS examinations performed. These are indicated to search for the underlying cause of dyspnea, particularly aspiration pneumonia, fluid overload, and/or pulmonary embolism, and to monitor the progression and/or resolution of any identifiable PLUS pathology over time.

MACHINE FUNCTIONS

Most PLUS clinical questions can be answered with confidence in the absence of obtaining the "perfect image", in a short amount of time and without using expensive or advanced ultrasound equipment. A portable, hand held, or refurbished ultrasound machine is sufficient for most PLUS applications. Things to consider in purchasing a machine include cost, mobility, resolution, start-up time, durability, and transducer selection. A mobile machine that can be brought to the patient, and a microconvex 5–8 MHz transducer, is sufficient for most POCUS applications, including PLUS. Although ultrasound units have multiple machine functions, there are only three main functions that are essential to understand in performing PLUS: gain, depth, and frequency (Fig. 1).

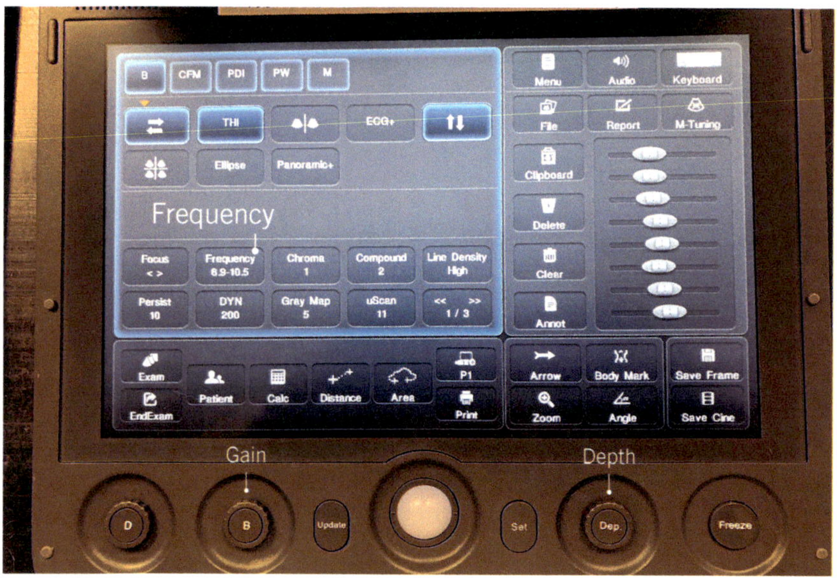

Figure 1. Typical ultrasound machine keyboard. The 3 main ultrasound machine functions used during POCUS examinations: gain, depth and frequency. The gain is used to make an image sharper and to highlight different structures and fluid. Depth is used to change how deep the ultrasound beams go and what is visible on the screen. The frequency setting of the transducer will affect image quality and depth perception.

- **Gain** controls the overall "brightness", making the image sharper to highlight different structures and pathology such as fluid. The "ideal" gain varies by operator; a general rule is for the operator to make the image "look pretty". For PLUS, gain is adjusted to visualize the pleural line and lung sliding (glide sign), keeping in mind the lung sliding is easier to visualize as the pleural line is made to look "grainier" (see Chapter 3). If the abdomen is scanned prior to PLUS, the gain will often need to be decreased as abdominal POCUS tends to use higher gain settings, which makes the pleural line overly hyperechoic and identification of lung sliding more challenging.
- **Depth** is used to change how deep the ultrasound beams go and what can be visualized in the ultrasound image. For PLUS, the pleural line should be located at a distance of roughly one-third of the total of the ultrasound image (depth is typically set at 2-6 cm for most PLUS scanning). Otherwise the depth should be adjusted to have the image or the organ of interest located at the top third to the middle of the ultrasound image. Too much depth will not allow visualization of key structures as they will appear too small. Not enough depth may result in the sonographer missing pathology below the organ or the area of interest. Most ultrasound machines indicate depth on one side of the ultrasound image, usually in centimeters, which can be used to estimate depth and size of structures in real time without having to use machine caliper functions for precise measurements.
- **Frequency** affects the image quality and depth perception. For PLUS scanning, frequencies used are usually in the range of 5–8 MHz. The higher the frequency, the more superficial the penetration of the ultrasound beam and the better the superficial quality of the image. Higher frequency settings will not allow visualization of deeper structures. The lower the frequency, the deeper the penetration of the ultrasound beam at the expense of decreasing image resolution. With most ultrasound transducers (especially microconvex curvilinear transducers), the frequency can be changed.

Knowledge and understanding of other ultrasound machine functions is helpful in specific situations but is not obligatory to the success of understanding and performing PLUS.

TRANSDUCER MANIPULATIONS

Acquisition of sonographic images involves manipulating the transducer and fine-tuning its position, in multiple directions, to display the ideal image. The smallest transducer movements (millimeters or even 1–2 degrees) can have a major impact on the plane in which the structure of interest is being scanned: it is often necessary to apply one transducer manipulation at a time, or the desired image may not be achieved. There are five key transducer movements used during PLUS: fanning, rocking, sweeping, sliding and rotating (Fig. 2). For descriptive purposes the part of the transducer that contacts the body surface is the "head" and the opposite end, where the

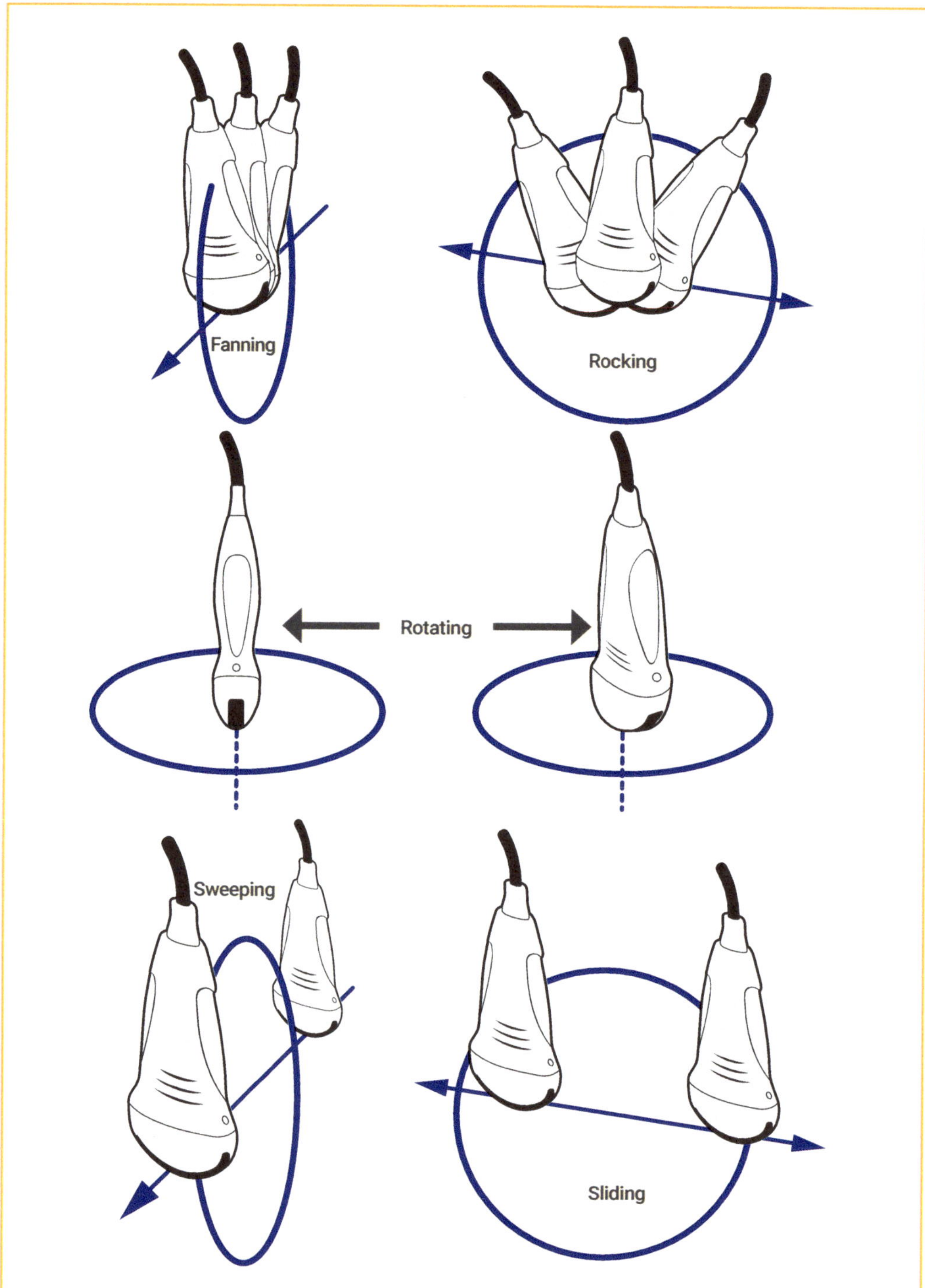

Figure 2. Transducer manipulations. Descriptive anatomy of the transducer with ultrasound beam angle of insonation.

Key transducer movements

- **Fanning** involves keeping the transducer head stationary and moving the tail of the transducer from side-to-side (changing the angle of insonation) relative to the transducer's widest axis, giving the impression of a "hand-held fan".
- **Rocking** the transducer involves keeping the transducer head stationary and moving the tail of the transducer from side-to-side (changing the angle of insonation) relative to the transducer's shortest axis (towards or away from the direction of the transducer marker), giving the impression of a "rocking chair".
- **Rotating** involves keeping the transducer head in one location perpendicular to the body surface, and turning the transducer upon its axis in a clockwise or counter-clockwise direction.
- **Sweeping** involves moving the entire transducer (usually a few centimetres) in the short axis direction across the body with a constant angle of insonation to the target.
- **Sliding** involves moving the entire transducer (usually a few centimetres) in the long axis direction across the body with a constant angle of insonation to the target.

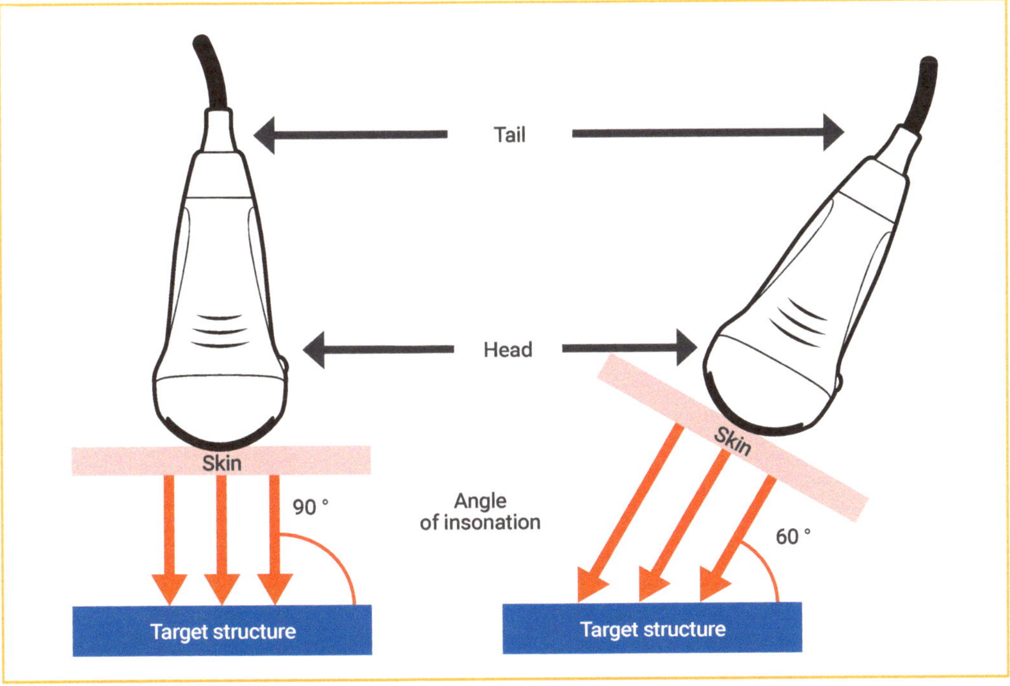

Figure 3. Transducer manipulations shown here as 90 degree and 60 degree angles of insonation to the target of interest.

cable attaches, is the "tail". The angle of the ultrasound beam relative to the organ of interest is referred to as the "angle of insonation" (Fig. 3).

When fanning, rocking or rotating, the transducer-to-body surface contact point remains the same, and the transducer is manipulated around the point of contact. With sweeping and sliding, the transducer head moves away from the initial point of contact on the body surface.

Transducer orientation

Each ultrasound transducer has an orientation marker (notch or depression) on one side which corresponds to a symbol or circle on the ultrasound image obtained on the screen (Fig. 4). This indicates transducer orientation (left or right on the screen) and provides a reference point which allows the transducer to be manipulated in such a way as to move the corresponding desired object of interest within the ultrasound image. Rocking and sliding manipulations will shift the image or move the desired object of interest within the image to the left or right.

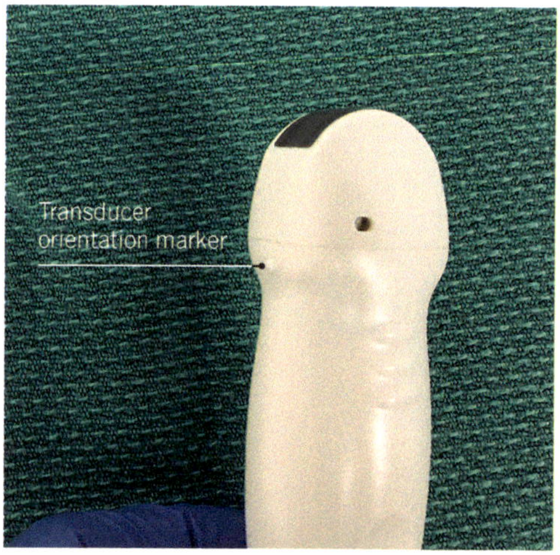

Figure 4. Ultrasound transducer (microconvex curvilinear) with an arrow indicating the marker on the transducer that allows for orientation of the image on the ultrasound machine. This marker correlates with a symbol, usually at the top right or left, of the ultrasound image produced.

Longitudinal (long) and transverse (short) axis

Longitudinal orientation describes placing the transducer in the "long" view (long axis) relative to the organ being evaluated (Fig. 5). Transverse orientation describes placing the transducer in the "short" view (short axis) relative to the organ being evaluated (transverse to the organ). Short axis is obtained by rotating the transducer 90 degrees from the long axis, often with the orientation marker directed dorsally (e.g. toward the spine) when the transducer is placed on the lateral surface of the patient (e.g. during lung or renal scanning), or with the orientation marker to the right of the patient if the transducer is placed on the ventral midline (e.g. scanning the liver in short axis).

PATIENT POSITIONING AND PREPARATION

The machine is brought to the patient, which can be in sternal recumbency or standing (preferred position for dyspneic patients), or in lateral recumbency (the latter is reserved for patients that are not in respiratory distress). Positioning in dorsal recumbency has the potential to decompensate patients with respiratory or cardiovascular compromise; for instance, the abdominal organs push on the diaphragm, which can cause increased respiratory effort in patients with pleura,

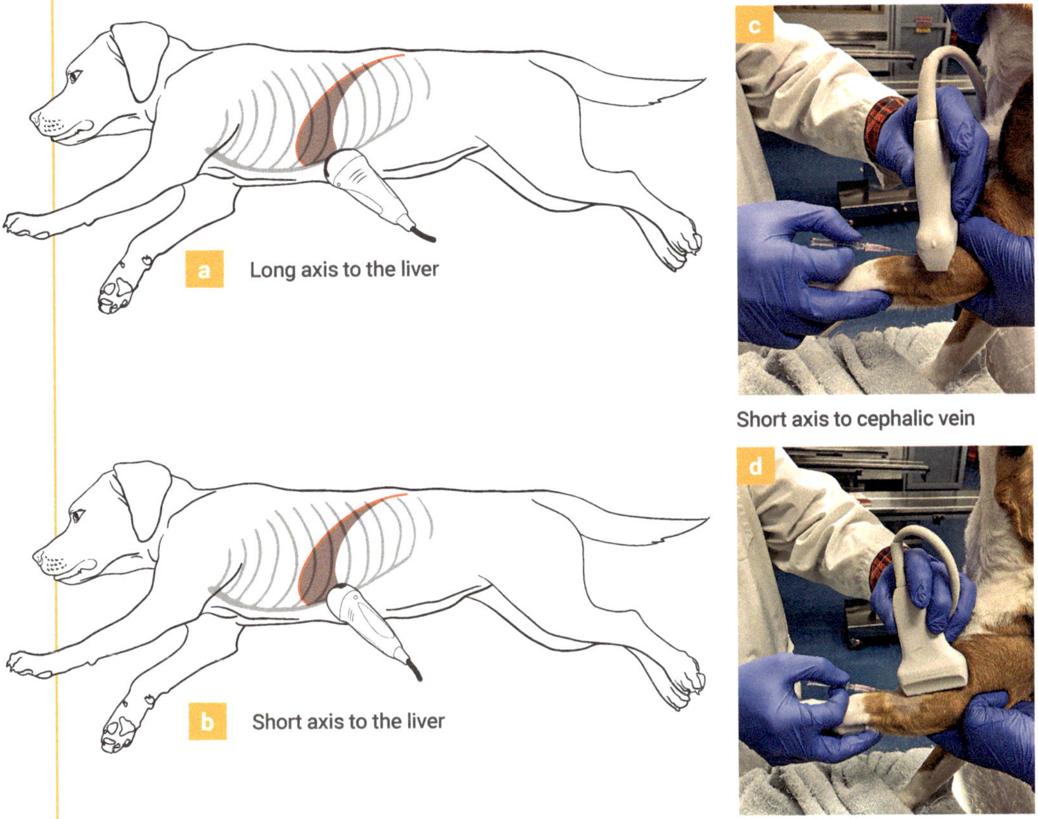

Figure 5. Longitudinal (long) (a) vs. transverse (short) axis (b). Long axis describes placing the transducer in the "long" view relative to the organ being evaluated with ultrasound whereas short axis is the "short" view (transverse to the organ). Short axis is obtained by rotating the transducer 90 degrees, often with the marker of the transducer towards the spine or dorsally when the transducer is placed on the lateral surface of the patient (e.g. during lung or renal scanning), or with the marker to the right of the patient if the transducer is placed on the ventral midline (e.g. scanning the liver in short axis). The pictures depict placing a cephalic IV catheter in short (c) and long (d) axis to the vein using a linear transducer. In long axis, the transducer is parallel to the vein whereas in short axis the transducer is perpendicular.

pleural space or lung pathology, and on the great vessels such as the caudal vena cava, decreasing venous return, which may cause cardiovascularly unstable patients to worsen. Shaving is generally not required, and alcohol is often used as the coupling agent. The fur is parted prior to application of alcohol to allow direct contact between the ultrasound transducer and skin surface, which improves image quality. Gel can be used in addition to alcohol, although care should be taken to avoid trapping air within the fur and gel. In patients with a thick undercoat clipping may improve image quality. Minimal

PLUS key points

- The accumulation of fluid and air within the pleural space are influenced by gravity, lung recoil and the anatomy of the pleural recesses. It is crucial to consider these factors, in light of patient positioning, to maximize the chance of detecting pathology.
- Defining sonographic pleura and lung borders on either side of the chest standardizes the areas scanned, regardless of species or breed differences, and ensures the most sensitive sites for pathology are evaluated.
- The abdominal curtain sign orientates the sonographer to the caudal thoracoabdominal border, which should be assessed for the presence of pneumothorax, pleural effusion and lung consolidation.
- The caudodorsal anatomic border is sonographically identified and assessed for pneumothorax in the standing/sternally recumbent patient.
- The ventral anatomic borders are sonographically identified and assessed for small-volume pleural effusion in the standing/sternally recumbent patient.
- Turning the transducer parallel to ribs in the ventral thoracic regions makes identification of the ventral pleural borders easier and assists in finding small volumes of pleural effusion.
- The pericardiodiaphragmatic window is assessed to help differentiate pleural from pericardial effusion.
- A sliding "S" pattern is used to ensure multiple lung regions are scanned in a rapid fashion.
- The subxiphoid site is also included.

to no restraint is required. Oxygen therapy and anxiolytics may help to calm dyspneic, tachypneic or anxious patients, decreasing the respiratory rate and effort, and making interpretation of PLUS findings easier, particularly lung sliding.

CALGARY PLUS APPROACH

A step-by-step general PLUS scanning approach is described below for the sternally recumbent or standing patient, emphasizing the identification of thoracic pleura and lung borders in a comprehensive, standardized and systematic manner (Fig. 6).

1. Place the transducer on a region of the thorax where lung can be reliably identified: behind the thoracic limb (the cranial PLUS border), roughly between the fifth and sixth intercostal spaces at the cranial thoracic border and half to two-thirds of the way up the thorax (Fig. 7; video 1). This ensures the transducer is placed over lung, avoids the heart and also avoids placing the transducer in areas other than the thorax such as the abdominal cavity, and misinterpreting findings such as gastric gas and peritoneal fluid as pathologic findings believed to be in the thorax.
2. The transducer is typically placed in a perpendicular orientation to the ribs (Fig. 8);

this positioning has the advantage of allowing the identification of the bat sign, (see Chapter 3), which helps in locating the pleural line.

3. Normal structures are then identified (see Chapter 3) and the pleural line is assessed for the presence or absence of lung sliding (Fig. 9) or the presence of pleural effusion (see Chapter 5).
4. If lung sliding is seen at the initial transducer location, the transducer should be slid caudally until the abdominal curtain sign is identified (thoracoabdominal interface; a sharp sonographic vertical demarcation depicting the transition from lung to soft tissue structures of the abdomen) (Fig. 10; see Chapter 3). Within the abdominal cavity, soft tissue organs will become visible (stomach, kidneys, liver, etc).

   Once the abdominal curtain sign has been identified and assessed, the transducer is slid caudodorsally along it until the hypaxial muscle–pleural space junction is identified (dorsal PLUS border; Fig. 11). This junction is identified by the loss of the pleural line when the transducer slides onto the hypaxial muscles. The transducer is slid ventrally again until the pleural line is once again just visible. This is the caudodorsal site of the thorax, and the area in which free pleural air is most likely to accumulate in cases of pneumothorax when patients are in a sternal or standing position (see Chapter 4).
   - If a lung sliding is seen here it is unlikely pneumothorax is present on that side of the thorax in the standing or sternal patient.
   - Note: to avoid confusing the abdominal curtain sign for lung sliding at the caudodorsal site, the transducer can be advanced a rib space cranial to the abdominal curtain sign. This allows lung sliding to be interpreted without the confusion of seeing a moving curtain sign.
   - If lung sliding is not seen at the most caudodorsal site, pneumothorax should be suspected and a search for the lung point or return of lung sliding undertaken (see Chapter 4).
5. If lung sliding was identified in step 4, the scan is continued by sliding the transducer across the intercostal spaces and over the thorax in an "S" shaped fashion. This allows multiple lung regions to be evaluated for lung pathology, and the ventral thoracic regions to be assessed for pleural effusion (Fig. 12).
   - From the transducer location in step 4, the transducer is slid across the dorsal third of the thorax as cranially as possible while continuing to visualize the pleural line for pathology (Fig. 13a).
   - The most cranial portion of the thorax that can be scanned is defined by the flexor muscles of the shoulder and the scapula.
   - If pathology is suspected, the transducer should be held stationary at that location to further confirm or refute the presence of pathology.
   - Once at the scapula/flexor muscles of the shoulder are encountered (the craniodorsal portion of the thorax), the transducer is slid ventrally within the cranial intercostal space until the midthoracic region is reached (base of the heart region; Fig. 13b).
   - The transducer is then slid caudally at the midthoracic level until the abdominal curtain sign is identified (Fig. 13c),

continuing to visualize the pleural line for pathology.

- Once the abdominal curtain sign is identified, the transducer is slid ventrally along it until the diaphragm and heart are visible in the same sonographic window. This is the pericardiodiaphragmatic window (caudoventral region of the thorax; Figs. 13d and 14a–b; see Chapter 3). Any pathology at the pericardiodiaphragmatic window is noted. Note that the heart and diaphragm can often be identified in the same window on the left and right side the chest in healthy dogs but are not always visible together in healthy cats.

  If present, pericardial effusion as well as large to moderate quantities of pleural effusion will be visible at the pericardiodiaphragmatic window. If pleural effusion is not visible at the pericardiodiaphragmatic window, the transducer should be rotated 90 degrees clockwise (marker dorsal; Fig. 14b) and then slid ventrally until the sternal muscles and lung or heart are both visible in the sonographic window (Fig. 15a–b). Scanning the ventral regions with the transducer parallel to the ribs and rocking the transducer increases the chance of detecting scant to small volumes of pleural effusion (see Chapter 5).
- From this location, maintaining a parallel transducer orientation to the ribs, the transducer is slid cranially an intercostal space at a time while searching for pleural effusion (Fig. 16).
- At the sixth to the fourth intercostal spaces, the heart may become visible adjacent to the sternal muscles (Fig. 15b).
- If the heart and sternal muscles are visible in the same sonographic window, sliding the transducer dorsally, from the sternal muscles across the heart, with the transducer still orientated parallel to the ribs, will encounter the ventral regions of the lung (regions where lung is often superimposed over the heart on thoracic radiographs).
- The transducer can be slid dorsal and ventral to the heart to assess for lung and pleural space pathology respectively, while also moving an intercostal space at a time cranially until the thoracic limb or thoracic inlet are encountered.

6. The other side of the thorax should be scanned in a similar fashion.
7. The subxiphoid area should also be included (Fig. 17). The transducer can be placed in long and short axis to the body in the subxiphoid region and the transducer rocked so that the ultrasound beams penetrate the thorax. Once the thorax is visualized, the transducer is fanned, through an angle of 45 degrees to either side of midline, and rocked to ensure adequate scanning of this region.
   - If the patient is standing, access to the subxiphoid region is gained by palpating the "V" of the subxiphoid region and placing the transducer in this location in both long and short axis (Fig. 18a). The transducer is then rocked and fanned so that the ultrasound beams penetrate the thorax, often by angling the transducer almost parallel to the spine.

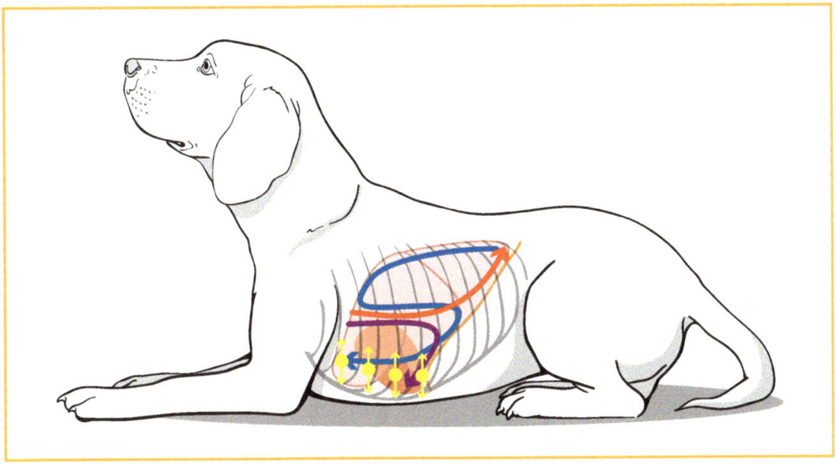

Figure 6. Calgary PLUS approach showing all systematic transthoracic scanning techniques that can be used to evaluate the pleural space and lung for various underlying pathologies. The red curved arrow describes how to make sure scanning starts over lung and then identifies the caudal (abdominal curtain sign) and dorsal PLUS borders (hypaxial muscles) of the thorax. This brings the transducer to the most sensitive area to rule out pneumothorax in a sternal/standing patient. The blue "S"-shaped arrow describes how to thoroughly scan the lungs to look for pathology. The yellow arrows describe transducer movements ventrally with the transducer in parallel orientation to the ribs to detect small amounts of pleural effusion. The purple arrow describes how to reach the pericardiodiaphragmatic region, to help differentiate pleural and pericardial effusion. Although not shown in this diagram, the subxiphoid window is also be included when performing PLUS. See following sections and Fig. 17a for how to modify the approach based on the presenting history and triage findings.

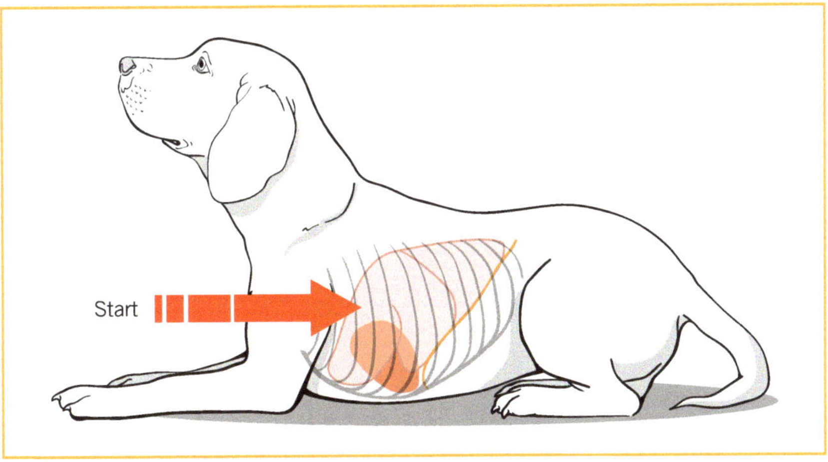

Figure 7. Initial transducer placement. The transducer should be on a region of the thorax where lung can be reliably identified, behind the thoracic limb, roughly between the 5th-6th intercostal spaces and 1/2 to 2/3rds of the way up the thorax. This avoids placing the transducer in areas other than the thorax such as the abdominal cavity, and misinterpreting findings such as gastric gas and peritoneal fluid as pathologic findings believed to be in the thorax.

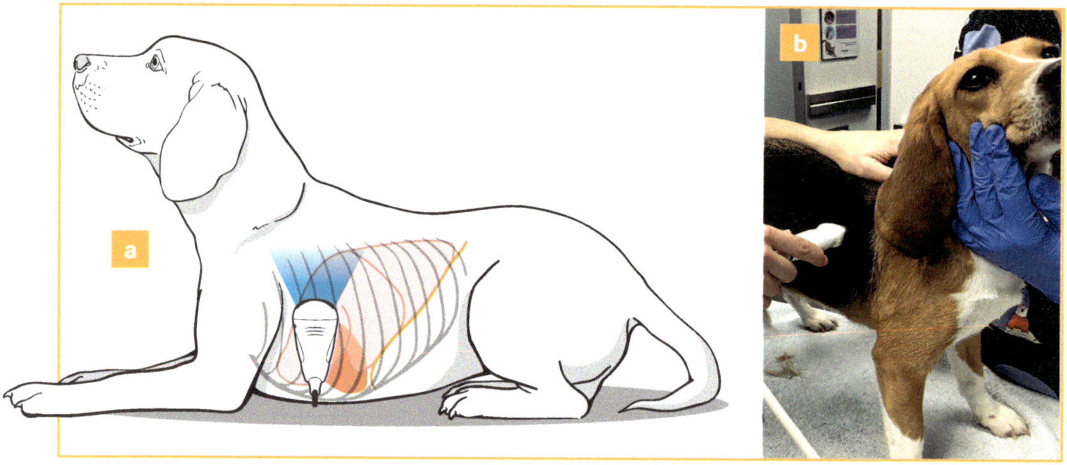

Figure 8. Schematic drawing of the transducer being placed perpendicular to the ribs, at the initial starting point (a). The advantage of placing the transducer in this fashion is to identify the bat sign, which helps in locating the pleural line, as well as making sure lung is observed (and not abdominal structures). Image of the transducer held perpendicular to the ribs of a dog (b). The head of the dog is to the right of the image, and the imagers left hand is at the thoracolumbar region. In this photo, the transducer has been slid caudally from the recommended starting point behind the scapula/flexor muscles of the shoulder and is located over the abdominal curtain sign about 2/3 of the way up the thorax.

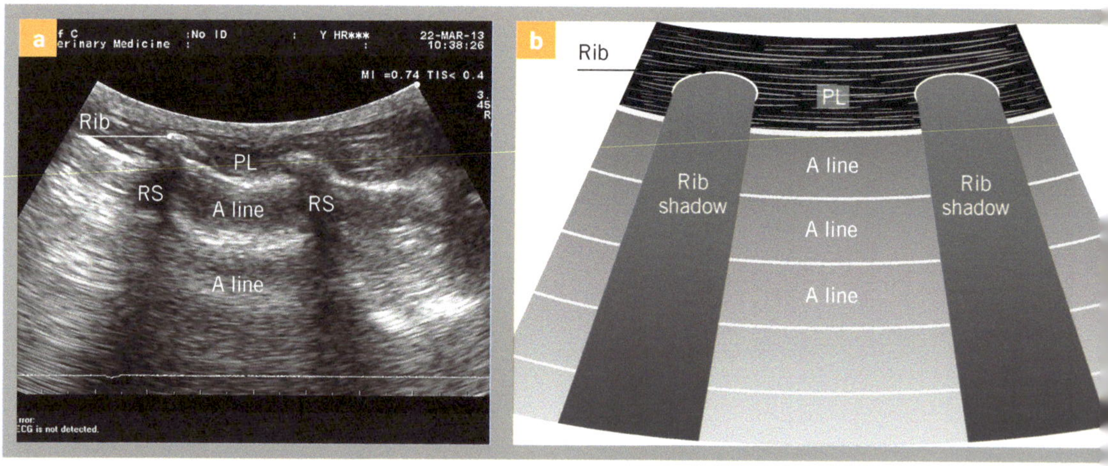

Figure 9. Labelled still ultrasound image when the transducer is placed perpendicular between two ribs (a). The pleural line is the first bright white line below the proximal rib surface that joins the rib shadows and in a normal dog or cat this line is the summation of the parietal and visceral pleura. Lung sliding is evaluated at the pleural line to determine if the two pleura are in contact. A lines are visible as horizontal white lines and are described in greater detail elsewhere. Schematic depicting the image obtained when the transducer is placed perpendicular between two ribs (b). RS; rib shadow, PL; pleural line.

If lung sliding (glide sign) is not seen at the initial transducer location, pneumothorax should be suspected and a search undertaken for the lung point, return of lung sliding, and/or abnormal curtain signs.

QR
Video 2.1.
Calgary PLUS approach.

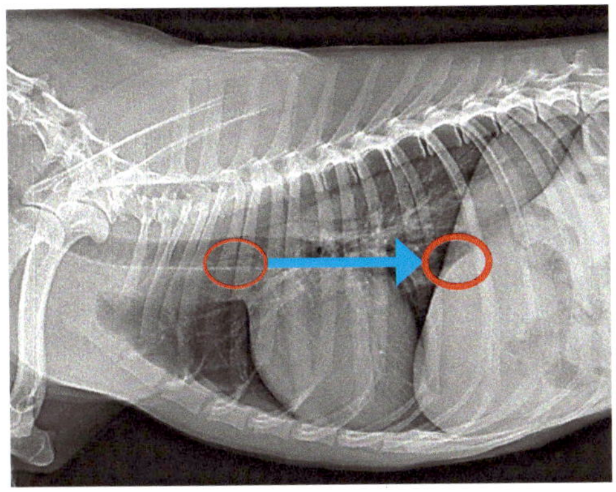

Figura 10. Finding the abdominal curtain sign (thoracoabdominal interface), lateral thoracic radiograph. From the initial starting point at cranial PLUS border (thin red circle), the transducer is slid caudally (blue arrow) between rib spaces until the abdominal curtain sign becomes visible (thick red circle), caudal PLUS border.

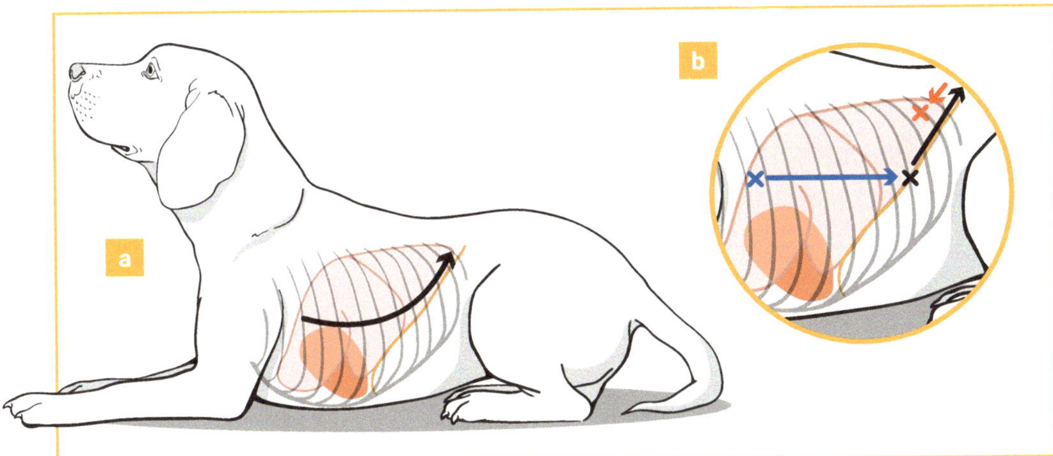

Figura 11. Finding the most caudodorsal area of the thorax in a standing/sternal patient. The curved black arrow demonstrates how the transducer is initially placed onto the thorax at the cranial PLUS border, slid to the abdominal curtain sign (caudal PLUS border), then slid in a slightly caudodorsal fashion to follow the abdominal curtain sign until lung sliding disappears and the hypaxial muscles are found (hypaxial muscle-pleural space junction), dorsal PLUS border (a). Further breakdown on where to initially place the transducer at the cranial PLUS border (blue X), sliding caudally (blue arrow) until the abdominal curtain sign is seen at the caudal PLUS border (black X), then sliding caudodorsal along the abdominal curtain sign until the pleural line is lost in the hypaxial muscles at the dorsal PLUS border (black arrow), followed by sliding ventrally (red arrow) until the pleural line is just visible again (red X) (b).

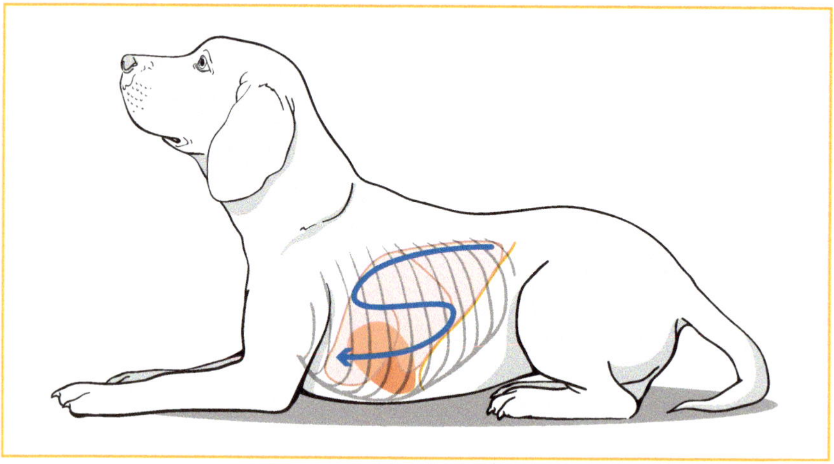

Figure 12. Scanning the thorax of a lateral patient in an "S" fashion (blue arrow) starting at the most caudodorsal site of the thorax.

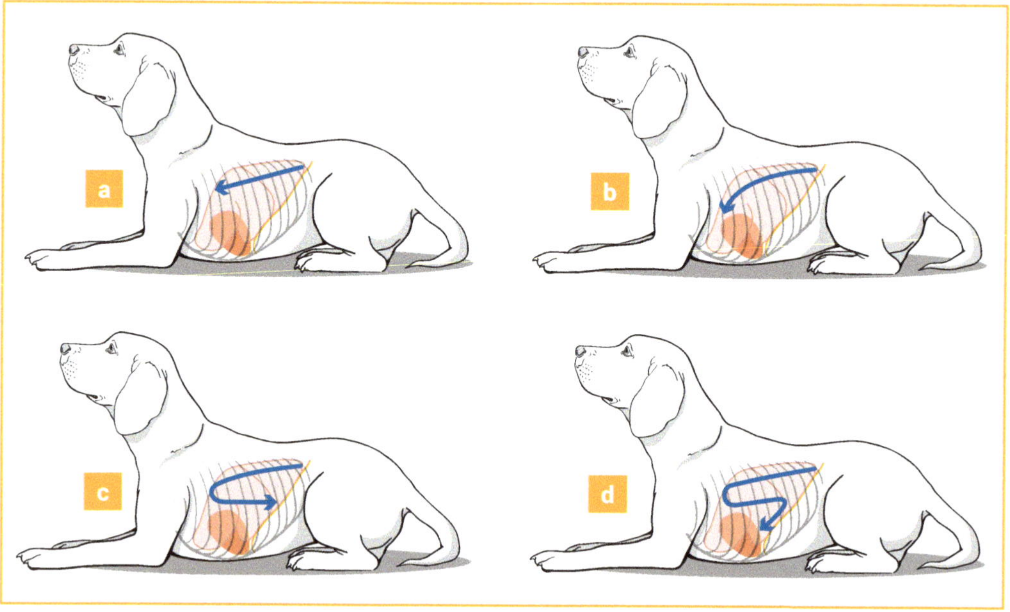

Figure 13. From the most caudal dorsal location, the transducer is slid across the dorsal 1/3 of the thorax as cranial as possible while continuing to visualize the pleural line for pathology (a). The most cranial portion of the thorax imaged will be at the caudal surface of the scapula and flexor muscles of the shoulder (cranial PLUS border). Once at the craniodorsal portion of the thorax, the transducer is slid ventrally to the mid-thorax (heart base region) (b) and then slid caudally towards the abdominal curtain sign (caudal PLUS border) while continuing to visualize the pleural line for pathology (c). Once the abdominal curtain sign is identified, the transducer is slid ventrally until the pericardiodiaphragmatic region (caudoventral region of the thorax) is identified and interrogated for pathology (d).

Figure 14. Thoracic radiograph illustration identifying the pericardiodiaphragmatic window of the thorax at the caudoventral border (a). This region is instrumental in differentiating pleural from pericardial effusion. If present, pericardial effusion, as well as large to moderate quantities of pleural effusion, will be visible at the pericardiodiaphragmatic window. When the transducer is turned parallel to the ribs, and then slid ventrally small amounts of pleural effusion, not visible with the transducer perpendicular to the ribs, are more easily identified (b).

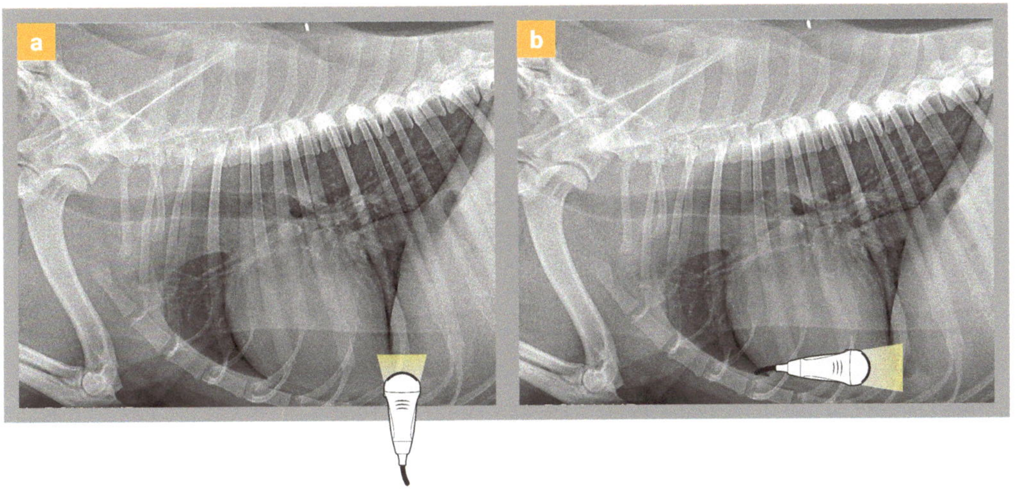

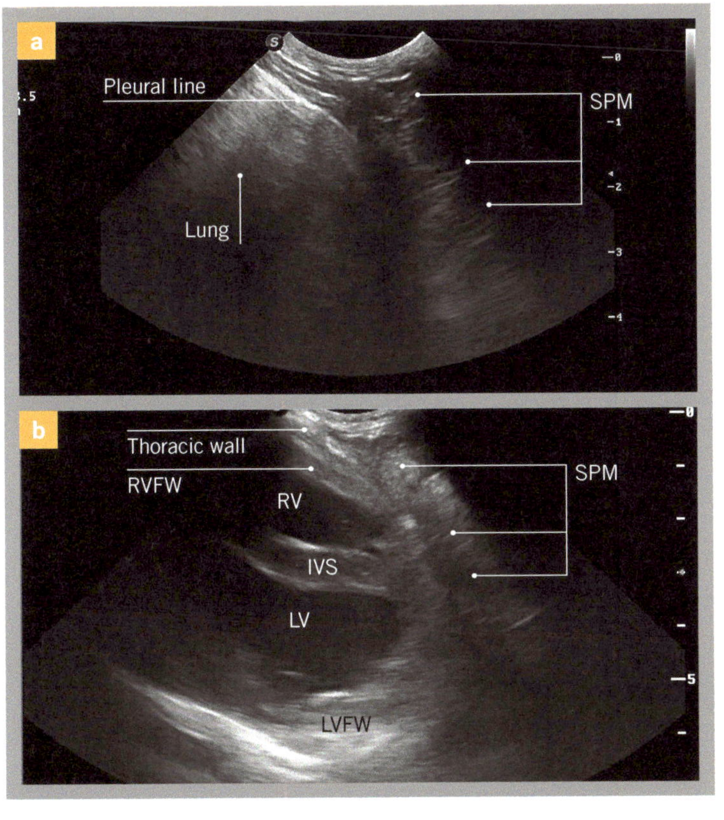

Figure 15. The most ventral regions of the thorax with the transducer orientated parallel to the ribs will visualize the lung sternal muscle interface or the heart sternal muscle interface. Ultrasound still image depicting the pleural line (parietal pleura visceral pleura interface), sternal muscles and lung with the transducer orientated parallel to the ribs in the ventral pleural region (a). Ultrasound still image depicting the interface between the heart and sternal/pectoral muscles with the transducer orientated parallel to the ribs at the most ventral regions (b). LV; left ventricle, RV; right ventricle, IVS; interventricular septum; RVFW; right ventricular free wall, LVFW; left ventricular free wall, SPM; sternal pectoral muscles.

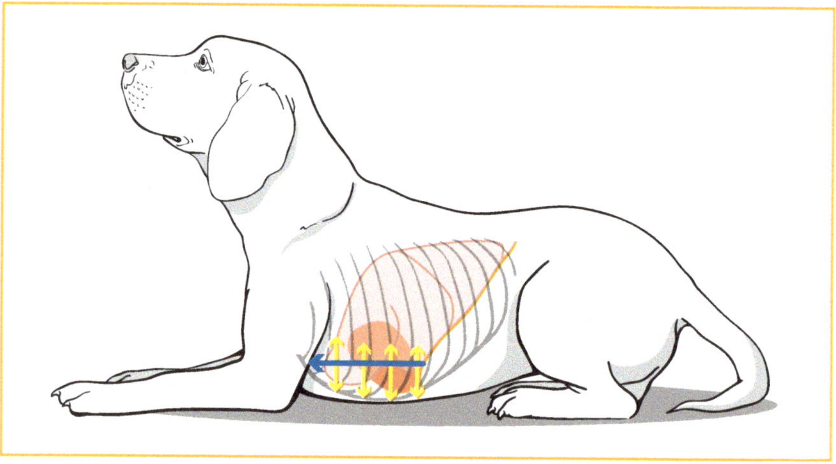

Figure 16. Turning the transducer to a parallel orientation to the ribs ventrally. Once at the ventral thoracic regions, the transducer can be turned parallel to the ribs (in between two ribs; yellow arrows) and slid ventrally a few centimetres until the sternal muscles are encountered to look for small amounts of pleural effusion at the ventral pleural PLUS border. Sliding the transducer a few centimetres dorsally after identifying the sternal muscles allows the ventral portions of the lungs to be assessed for pathology. The transducer should be slid cranially a rib space at a time, maintaining a parallel orientation to the ribs, until the thoracic inlet is encountered (blue arrow).

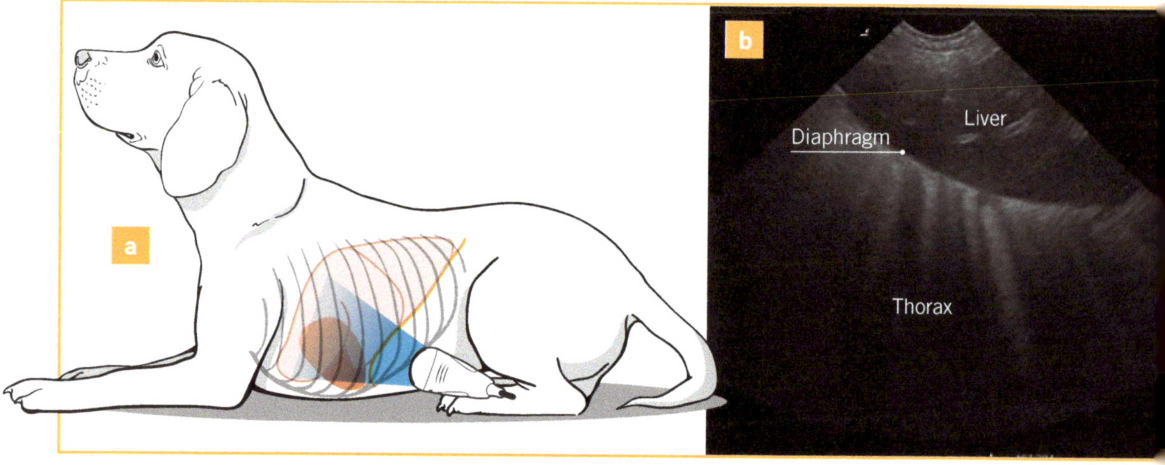

Figure 17. Subxiphoid site to evaluate the pleural space and lung. The transducer can initially be placed in long axis to the body in the subxiphoid region and the transducer rocked so that the ultrasound beams penetrate the thorax (a). Once the thorax is visualized, the transducer is fanned to ensure adequate scanning of this region. Still image obtained from the subxiphoid view depicting the liver, diaphragm and pleural space/lung beyond the diaphragm (b). Multiple B-lines can be seen radiating from the diaphragm in this image (see Chapter 3).

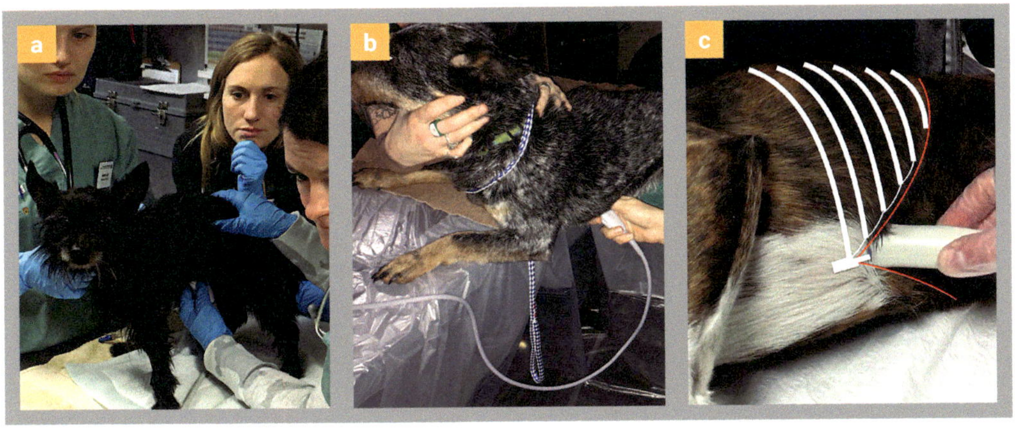

Figure 18. If the patient is standing (a), gaining access to the subxiphoid region is achieved by palpating the "V" of the subxiphoid region and placing the transducer in this location in both long and short axis. The transducer is then rocked and fanned so that the ultrasound beams penetrate the thorax, often by angling the transducer almost parallel to the body. If the patient is in sternal recumbency (b), the subxiphoid region can be accessed by placing two tables in an "L" fashion and lying the patient's subxiphoid region in the gap formed by the two tables. If the patient is in lateral recumbency the subxiphoid site is easily identified by tracing the ribs cranially and placing the transducer just caudal to the xiphoid process (c).

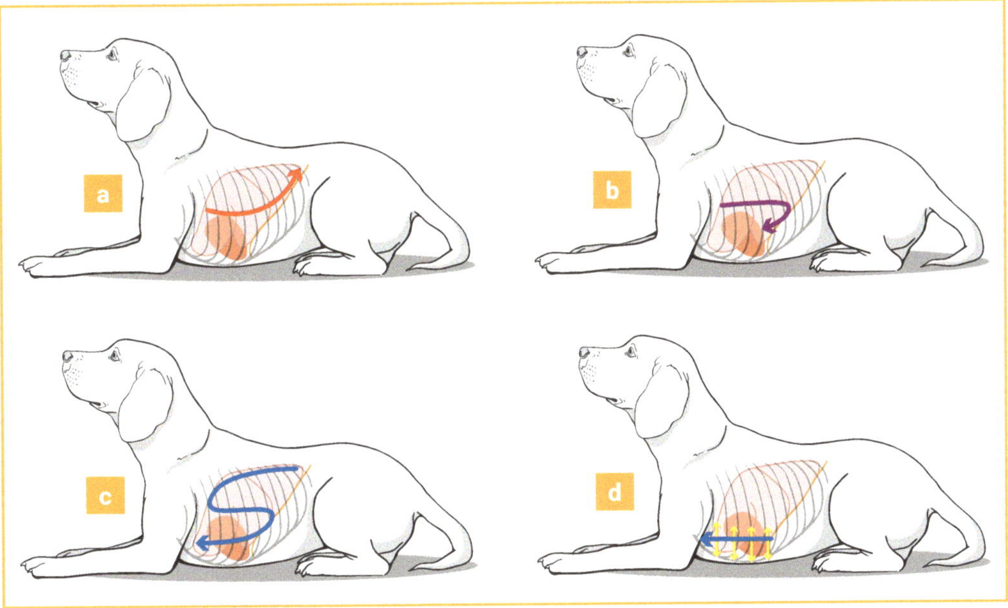

Figure 19. Overview of the PLUS approach in a sternal patient. The red arrow shows the initial transducer placement at the cranial PLUS border and movements to reach the most caudodorsal portions of the thorax (a). The purple arrow shows the starting point to reach the pericardiodiaphragmatic window (b). The blue arrow shows the "S" fashion sliding of the transducer to scan multiple regions of the lung in a systematic and rapid fashion to look for pathology (c). The yellow arrows indicate how the transducer can be turned in a parallel fashion to identify smaller amounts of pleural effusion. Although not shown in these diagrams, the subxiphoid window is also included when performing PLUS. The majority of the thorax with emphasis on its borders are scanned with this protocol (d).

- If the patient is in sternal recumbency, the subxiphoid region can be accessed by placing two tables in an "L" fashion and lying the patient's subxiphoid region in the gap formed by the two tables (Fig. 18b).
- If the patient is in lateral recumbency, the subxiphoid can be easily reached and palpated. The transducer can be placed in this region in both long (Fig. 18c) and short axis.

APPLICATION OF THE CALGARY PLUS APPROACH

Although much of the current evidence for POCUS is adapted from the human literature, new research is rapidly being published that helps support and adapt POCUS of the pleural space and lung specifically to veterinary patients which, along with other well-established imaging modalities, makes PLUS very practical.

As described in Chapter 1, POCUS exams are applied differently depending on patient history and clinical findings. In the emergency setting, limited triage examination and the minimum emergency database allow for rapid patient assessment in an attempt to identify life-threatening pathology and direct immediate therapeutic and additional diagnostic testing.

The same principle applies to PLUS in the emergency setting. Figs. 19 and 20 describe how initial triage examination findings dictate the specific binary PLUS question asked, and in what order the PLUS scan should initially be conducted to quickly identify patient pathology and gain rapid insight into immediate therapeutic and diagnostic interventions. For example, if history and triage examination suggests pneumothorax in a dyspneic patient, PLUS is applied to rule this in or out first: The transducer is slid from the starting point (step 1 of the PLUS protocol) to the abdominal curtain sign (step 3 for identifying normal abdominal curtain sign, see Chapter 3). If the abdominal curtain sign rules in pneumothorax (See Chapter 4) the patient is stabilized via thoracentesis and the remaining PLUS examination and other POCUS scans are completed when the patient is more stable. If the abdominal curtain sign is normal, the transducer is rapidly slid to the most caudodorsal border of the thorax to assess for a lung sliding (step 4; lung sliding rules out pneumothorax; see Chapter 4). If lung sliding is absent caudodorsally thoracentesis is performed to stabilize the patient, or a search for the lung point is undertaken to definitively rule in pneumothorax (see Chapter 4). If history and triage examination suggest pleural effusion is the main binary question to answer first, then the transducer is slid from its initial starting point (step 1) caudoventrally to assess the pericardiodiaphragmatic region, as well as scanning with the transducer turned parallel to the ribs ("sail" sign vs. "ski" jump; see Chapter 5). If the binary question centers on finding lung pathology, the transducer is slid from the starting position (step 1) to the most caudodorsal position and then across the thorax in an "S" fashion (step 5). The pathologies identified are discussed in subsequent chapters.

SUMMARY

Patient positioning, anatomic differences between species and breeds, mechanics of breathing, and the effects of gravity all affect where pleura and lung pathology localize, making these important factors to consider when performing PLUS. Sonographically identifying pleura and lung borders maximizes the detection of pathology in a standardized, repeatable, and systematic fashion. Clinically driven, often binary questions derived from the initial patient evaluation allow the application of a tailored PLUS scanning approach to rule pathology in or out in an efficient manner, followed by more comprehensive POCUS scanning when patients are more stable.

Figure 20. Use of Calgary PLUS for triage of unstable dyspneic patients.

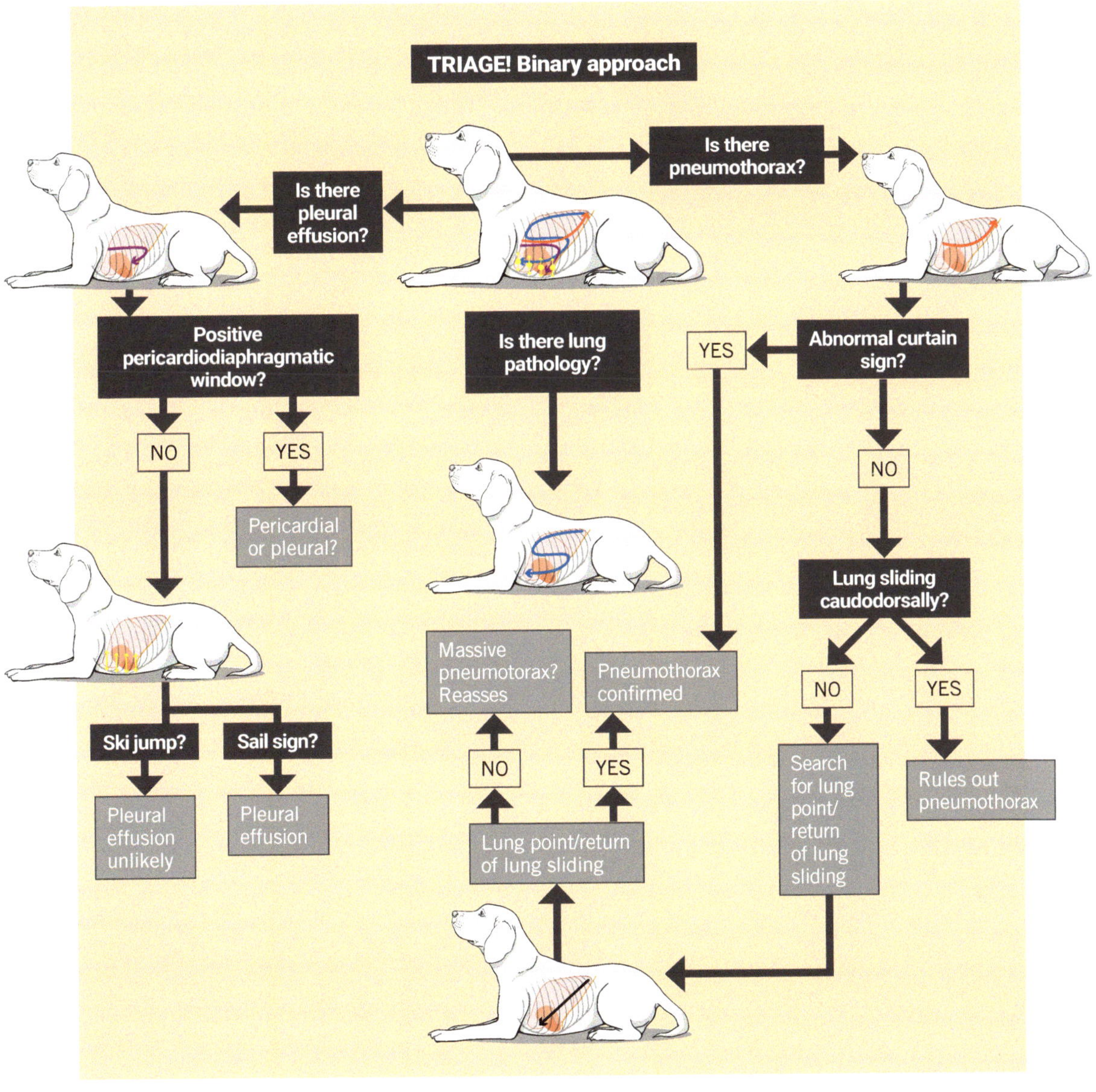

03

PLUS IMAGE INTERPRETATION: NORMAL FINDINGS

GENERAL PRINCIPLES

Pleura and lung ultrasound (PLUS) involves an understanding of how to interpret artifacts because healthy lungs contain air which impedes ultrasound transmission, rendering it impossible to visualize the lung itself. Fortunately, the normal findings of PLUS change because of underlying pleura and lung pathology, which allows identification of this pathology via artifact interpretation with relatively high sensitivity and specificity[1,2].

There are six key "lines and signs" to identify and interpret during PLUS:

1. Pleural line
2. A lines
3. Bat sign
4. Lung sliding (Glide sign)
5. B lines
6. Abdominal curtain sign.

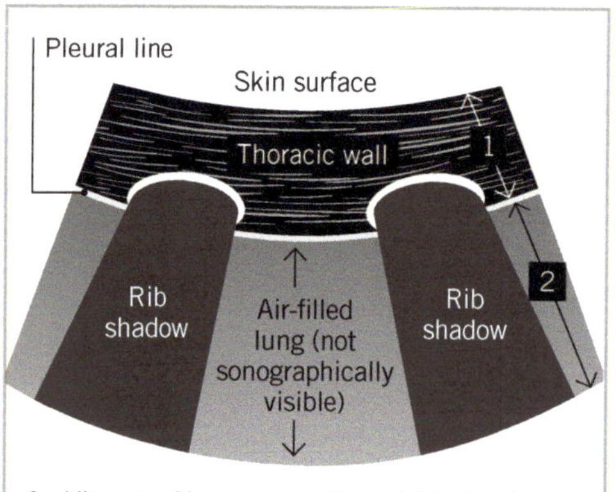

Figure 1. Schematic images of normal findings with a microconvex transducer placed transverse to the ribs over healthy lung.

In addition, knowing how to define dry lung and identify the pericardiodiaphragmatic (PD) window, the "ski jump" sign, the lung pulse, Z lines, I lines, and the five sonographically-defined pleura and lung borders (see Chapter 1) is also important when applying the Calgary PLUS approach.

When the transducer is placed transverse (perpendicular) to the ribs over the lungs, the ultrasound beam transmits through the soft tissue structures of the thoracic wall (skin, subcutaneous tissue, muscle layers) and encounters either bone or air, the two key enemies of PLUS (Fig. 1).

The two enemies of PLUS

Understanding the enemies of ultrasound is advantageous as they provide landmarks that allow the sonographer to identify key anatomic structures:

1. Bone: the ultrasound beam is attenuated and absorbed by bone, creating an anechoic black shadow which arises from and extends distal to the bone surface.
2. Air: the interface between soft tissue (thoracic wall) and air (e.g. air-filled lung or pneumothorax) reflects the vast majority of the ultrasound beam which creates a reverberation artifact below this interface.

If the ribs and rib shadows can be identified, the first continuous horizontal bright white line below the proximal rib surface that joins the rib shadows is the pleural line (Figs. 1 and 2).

THE PLEURAL LINE

Reflection of an ultrasound beam occurs at the interface between tissues with different acoustic impedance[1]. Given the low density of air, the difference in acoustic impedance between soft tissues and air is large, which produces hyperechoic images at the interface of reflection. This gives rise to the "bright white" pleural line. In healthy animals, the pleural line is a thin, smooth, relatively straight horizontal hyperechoic white line located just below the ribs joining the rib shadows, which is comprised of the parietal and visceral pleura (Fig. 2). The shape of the pleural line varies from straight to slightly curvilinear depending on the orientation of the ultrasound transducer, the type of transducer used and the shape of the thorax. A microconvex transducer generally produces a curvilinear pleural line compared to a linear transducer.

Anatomically speaking, the parietal and visceral pleura are two distinct sheets that are separated by a very small quantity of pleural fluid in healthy animals (Fig. 2a). Sonographically speaking, it is not possible to differentiate the two pleural sheets from each other or to visualize the scant quantity of pleural fluid between them in healthy patients. Instead, the two pleura are visualized as a single superimposed hyperechoic white line (Fig. 2b).

Although the appearance is sonographically identical on a still image, the pleural line can be comprised of both the parietal and visceral pleura when the lung surface is in contact with the thoracic wall or just the parietal pleura when the lung surface is separated from the thoracic wall. Separation of the pleura most often occurs because of pleural effusion, pneumothorax, and space-occupying soft tissue structures (e.g. foreign bodies, diaphragmatic hernia, neoplasia, etc). It is therefore essential to assess the pleural line carefully to determine if the two pleura are in contact or separated, which may be done directly through visualisation of the two pleura when they are separated by fluid or soft tissue structures, or indirectly

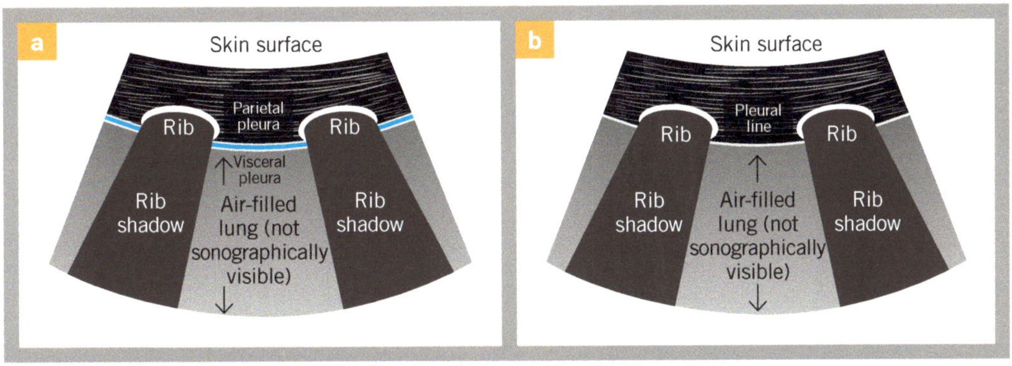

Figure 2. Anatomic and sonographic schematic images of healthy lung. Anatomical image depicting air filled lung (not sonographically visible) below the visceral pleura which is separated from the parietal pleural by a scant quantity of pleural fluid (shown in blue) (a). Sonographic image showing the two pleura (parietal and visceral) superimposed over each other, forming a single white line (pleural line) (b). The pleural fluid normally present in healthy animals is not visible on ultrasound.

through assessment of sonographic findings that suggest the two pleura are in contact and superimposed despite not seeing them directly (e.g. lung sliding, lung pulse, B lines).

The pleural line may vary in appearance if the soft tissue-to-air interface is lost, typically becoming less discernible. For example, when lung consolidations reach the lung surface the pleural line often becomes less hyperechoic over the site of consolidation as the soft tissue-to-air interface is replaced by a soft tissue-to-consolidation interface (see Chapter 7).

The pleural line is essential to identify as correct interpretation of artifacts arising from this line allow for the sonographic diagnosis of many pleura, pleural space and lung diseases.

A LINES

A lines are a type of reverberation artifact that result from the ultrasound beam being reflected back and forth between two highly reflective parallel surfaces: the soft tissue-to-air interface occurring at the pleural line and the skin–transducer interface. More than 99 % of the ultrasound beam is reflected from the pleural line and returns to the transducer (which registers a white line as the pleural line [Fig. 3a])[1]. The transducer reflects some of the returning ultrasound beam back towards the pleural line, which again reflects the ultrasound beam back to the transducer (Fig. 3). The ultrasound beam takes twice as long to return to the transducer the second time, which registers a "mirror" of the pleural line more distally on the ultrasound image, equidistant from the skin to pleural line. This is an A line.

Because A lines are the result of ultrasound beam reflection between the transducer and pleural line, they have the same shape as the pleural line. They are projected as horizontal white lines equidistant from the skin surface to the pleural line, tending to fade through the far field of the ultrasound image (Fig. 4).

Highly reflective structures (e.g. fascia, vessel walls, etc) located between the skin–transducer interface and the pleural line can also be repeatedly "mirrored" equidistant below the pleural line, similar to A lines. These "mirrored" structures should not be confused for lung pathology.

Because A lines require a soft tissue-to-air interface to be created, they are seen when aerated lung or pneumothorax occupies the region below the pleural line, and they will disappear when the normal soft tissue-to-air interface at the pleural line is lost. Their appearance will vary depending on the angle the ultrasound beam strikes the pleural line (Fig. 5). Therefore if A lines are not visible, it is important to ask if it is because of a narrow angle of insonation (weak echo) or because of a loss of the soft tissue-to-air interface (i.e. coalescent B lines, consolidations, pleural effusion, or pleural space occupying soft tissue structures are present below the pleural line).

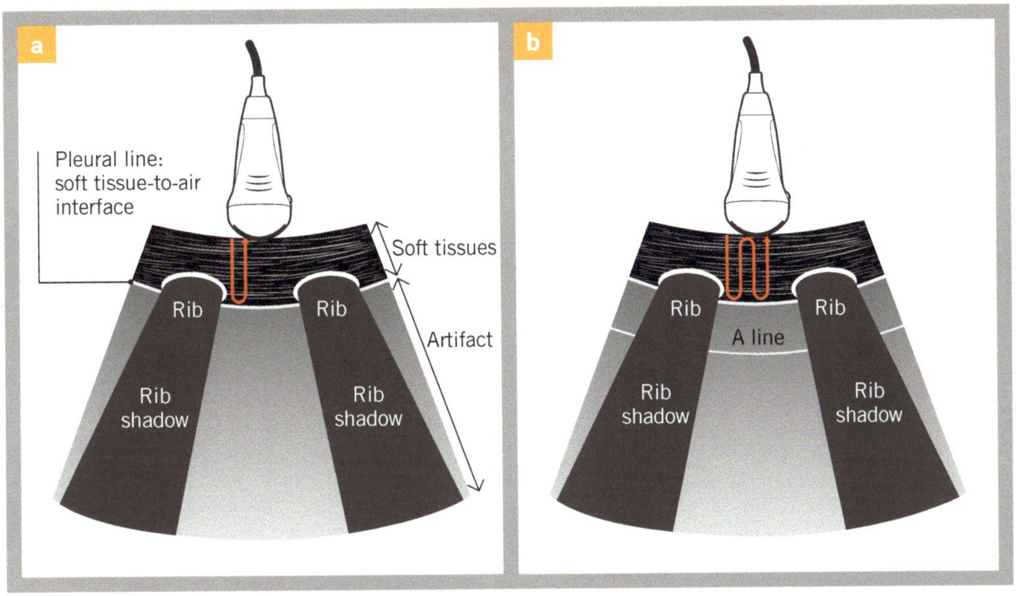

Figure 3. Schematic ultrasound images depicting the creation of A lines. The ultrasound beam (red curved arrow) travels from the transducer through the soft tissues of the thoracic wall to the soft tissue-to-air interface (in this example, aerated lung of a healthy animal). The ultrasound beam is reflected at the soft tissue-to-air interface and returns to the ultrasound transducer and a horizontal white line (pleural line) is registered on the ultrasound image (a). The ultrasound transducer reflects some of the returning ultrasound beam back towards the pleural line, which again reflects the ultrasound beam back to the transducer. The ultrasound beam takes twice as long to get back to the transducer, which registers a "mirror" of the pleural line more distally on the ultrasound image, equidistant from the skin to pleural line, which appears as an A line (b).

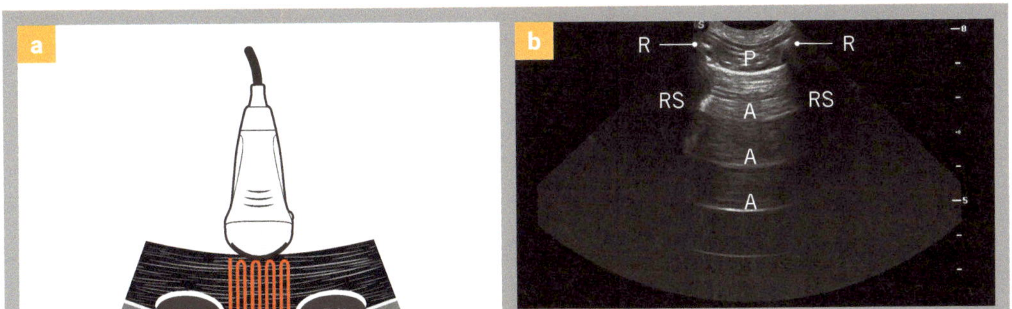

Figure 4. Schematic and still ultrasound image showing the presence of A lines. The ultrasound beam (red curved arrow) travels back and forth between the pleural line and transducer, creating multiple equidistant A lines through the far field image each time the beam returns to the transducer. A lines get fainter within the far field (a). Still ultrasound image taken from a healthy 3-year-old male Beagle dog demonstrating the fading of A lines (b). P; pleural line, A; A line, R; rib, RS; rib shadow.

Key points of the A lines:

A lines are present in healthy air-filled lung and cases of pneumothorax.

- They disappear when the soft tissue-to-air interface of the pleural line is lost due to:
  - Pleural effusion
  - Coalescent B lines
  - Consolidated lung
  - Pleural space occupying soft tissue structures

Their appearance changes depending on the angle of insonation at which the ultrasound beam strikes the pleura (Fig. 5):

- When the ultrasound beam is 90 degrees to the pleura (transducer head is parallel to the pleura), more of the ultrasound beam is reflected back and forth between the transducer and the pleura, resulting in a brighter pleural line and more visible A lines (strong echo; Figs. 5a and c).
- When the angle of insonation is decreased from 90 degrees (by fanning or rocking the transducer), less of the ultrasound beam is reflected back and forth between the transducer and the pleura, making the pleura appear "grainier" and A lines less visible (weak echo; Figs. 5b and d).
- If A lines are not visible, it is important to ask if it is because of the angle of insonation or because of a loss of the soft tissue-to-air interface (e.g. A lines are lost when lung consolidation is present just below the lung surface; see Chapter 7).

THE BAT SIGN

The bat sign, composed of the wings and body of a bat, is an imaginary aid to help sonographers orientate themselves to the key structures when a microconvex transducer is placed over the lung in a transverse orientation to the ribs (Fig. 6).

The bat sign is composed of:

- The proximal rib surfaces (ribs) which make up the wings of the bat (short white horizontal convex lines).
- The pleural line which makes up the body of the bat.

It is sometimes easier to identify and follow the rib shadows (black vertical artifact) proximally to the rib in order to find the wings of the bat. Once the wings are identified, the first horizontal white line below the ribs that joins the rib shadows should be identified: this is the body of the bat which signifies the pleural line. The pleural line is extremely important to identify as PLUS pathology results in sonographic changes arising from the pleural line (i.e. pleural fluid, absent lung sliding or a variety of artifacts).

The bat sign is sometimes referred to as the gator sign, however, the term bat sign is preferred as the letters help to identify the key features using mnemonics.

The ultrasound beam will not traverse Bone or Air when the transducer is orientated Transverse to the ribs (aka the BAT sign).

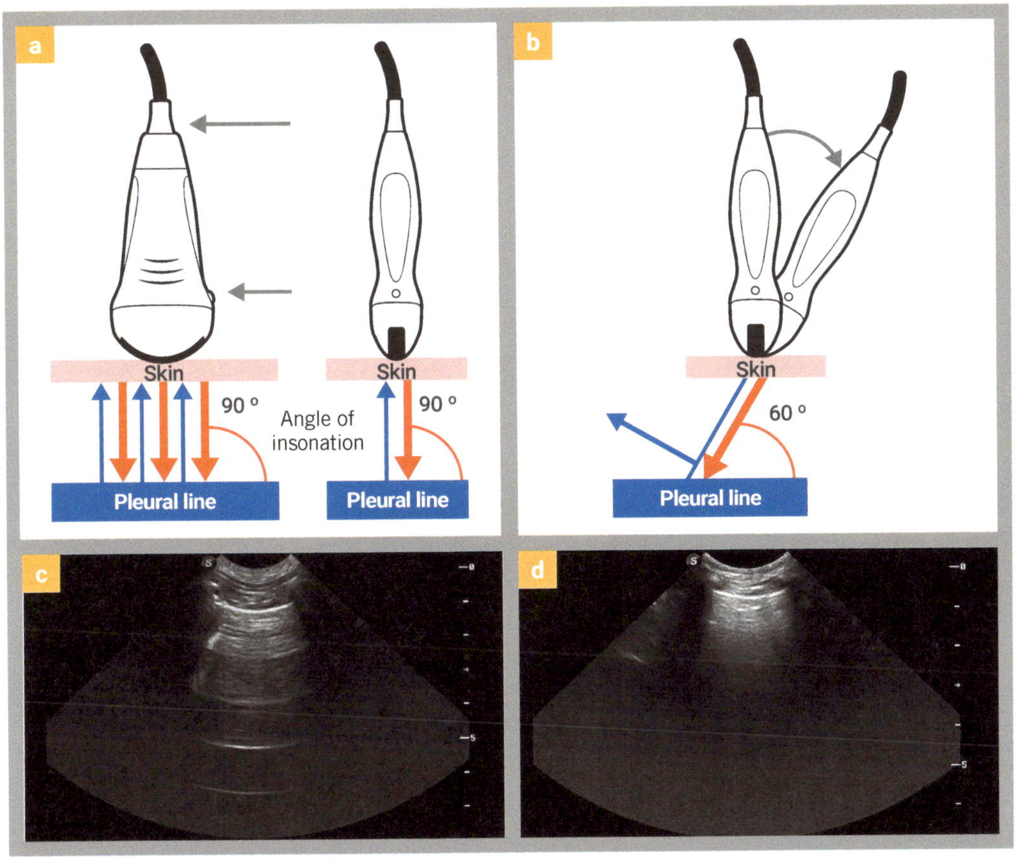

Figure 5. Schematic images depicting the angle of insonation the ultrasound beam encounters the pleura and the subsequent appearance of the pleural line and A lines (top), and their corresponding ultrasound still images obtained from a healthy 5-year-old mix-breed dog at the exact same site on the thorax (bottom). When the transducer surface is parallel to the pleura, the ultrasound beam strikes the pleura at a more perpendicular angle and most of the beam is reflected back and forth (blue and red arrows) between the transducer and soft tissue-to-air interface (pleural line), making the pleural line appear brighter and A lines become more visible (strong echo) (a). When the angle of insonation is decreased from perpendicular by fanning (shown) or rocking the transducer (not shown), the pleural line becomes less bright and A lines become less visible and may even disappear (weak echo) (b). The pleural line is brighter and A lines more visible as the transducer surface is parallel to the pleural line (c). The pleural line is not as bright and A lines are not visible at all (d).

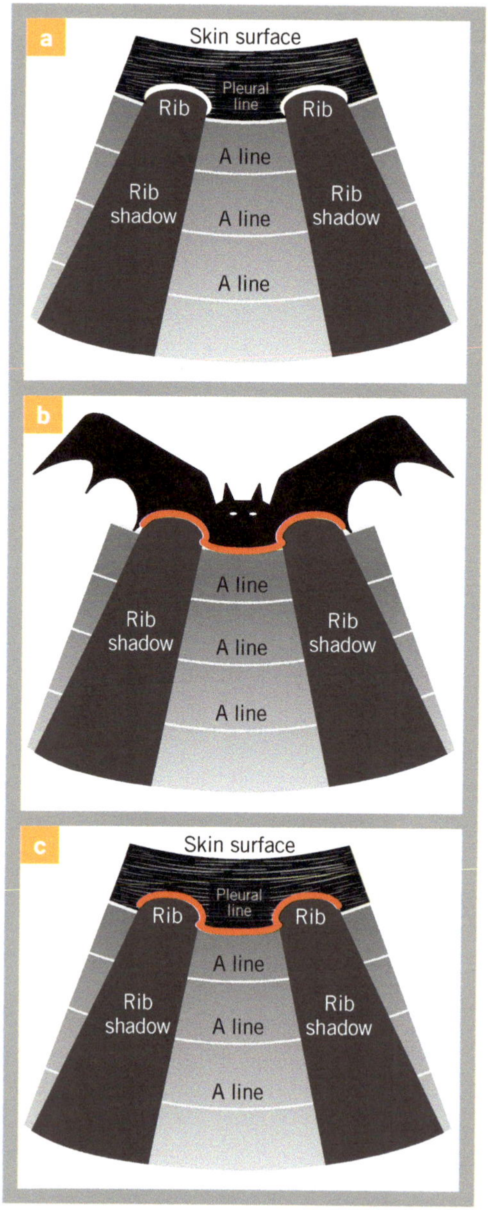

Figure 6. Schematic ultrasound image obtained with the microconvex transducer orientated transverse to the ribs showing the proximal rib surface, pleural line, rib shadows and A lines (a). The bat sign, which allows bone and air to be identified with the transducer transverse to the ribs helps sonographers to identify the pleural line (b). Representative wings and body of the bat with the actual bat removed for clarity (c).

LUNG SLIDING (THE GLIDE SIGN)

Lung sliding, also referred to as the "glide sign", is the to-and-fro shimmering along the pleural line which occurs as a result of the lung surface sliding along the thoracic wall during the respiratory cycle (video 3.1). When the patient inspires, the diaphragm contracts while the thoracic wall and parietal pleura expand outward. This subsequently results in lung expansion and causes the visceral pleura to slide along the internal thoracic wall. It is the movement of the two pleura sliding across each other at different speeds and in different directions that creates the visible shimmer of lung sliding (Fig. 7). The longer the distance the lungs slide across the thoracic wall (deep slow respirations), the easier it is to see lung sliding. Lung sliding is difficult to appreciate in patients that are panting or have shallow rapid respirations.

QR
Video 3.1. Lung slide.

The lungs tend to expand more in the caudodorsal regions of the thorax compared to the ventral regions, often making it easier to identify lung sliding caudodorsally than cranioventrally. In theory it should be possible to identify lung sliding over all sonographically-visible lung regions of healthy patients where the visceral and parietal pleura are in contact, although it may not be easy to appreciate at all sites. It may also be difficult to visualize lung sliding across the entire pleural line within a sonographic window of healthy animals, despite the pleura being in contact. This may lead to confusion in differentiating pleura that are in contact with difficult to visualize lung sliding from pleura that are separated due to pneumothorax and/or have a partial or intermittent lung slide visible at the lung point (see Chapter 4). Failure to differentiate partial or intermittent lung sliding associated with the lung point from lung sliding can lead the operator to mistakenly rule out pneumothorax, when the lung point actually confirms its presence (see Chapter 4)[3].

The key to identify lung sliding is to focus the eyes on the pleural line and ignore other distractions such as thoracic wall movements. The sonographer's hand and the patient must be kept as stationary as possible. Their movement makes interpretation of lung sliding more challenging and may create false positive lung sliding.

Visualization of lung sliding

As stated above, lung sliding is a dynamic finding and therefore only valid when the patient breathes, causing the lung to slide along the thoracic wall with the respiratory cycle. Unfortunately, lung sliding is not always easy to identify, even in healthy individuals, and becomes even harder to identify in patients with respiratory distress, pneumonia, rapid shallow breathing and patients that are panting[2,4]. Stabilizing the patient and providing oxygen and anxiolytics may decrease the respiratory rate making lung sliding easier to identify.

Lung sliding is often easier to identify if the pleural line is made "granier".

Pearls and considerations

There are two criteria for lung sliding to be sonographically visible:

- The visceral pleura must be in contact with the parietal pleura.
- The patient must breathe; the two pleura must slide across each other to create sonographically-visible shimmering.

Therefore lung sliding is absent when:

- The two pleura are not directly opposed (see Chapters 4 and 5).
  - Pleural separation can occur as a result of pleural effusion, pneumothorax and pleural space occupying soft tissue structures.
  - The two pleura are adhered to one another (e.g. pleural fibrosis).
  - Lung consolidation is present (see Chapter 6).
  - There is an absence of respiration.

Lung sliding is often present but reduced with low tidal volumes and cases with hyperinflated lungs (e.g. feline asthma), or difficult to appreciate in panting or dyspneic patients.

Lung sliding should be complete and visible across the entire pleural line in healthy animals, although it may be difficult to appreciate.

There are several tricks to make the pleural line appear "granier" and lung sliding easier to visualize:

- Change the angle the ultrasound beams strike the pleural line by fanning the transducer; the ultrasound beams strike the pleural line obliquely and not perpendicular

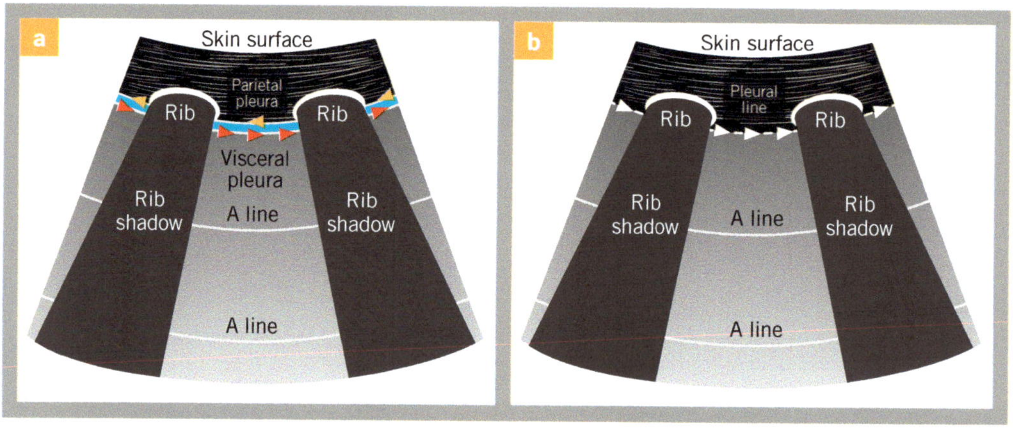

Figure 7. Schematic anatomical image during inspiration demonstrating the smaller movement of the parietal pleura (yellow arrow heads) relative to the larger movement of the visceral pleura (red arrow heads) which creates lung sliding. The two pleura are shown separated by a small quantity of pleural fluid which is not sonographically visible in healthy animals, and acts to prevent friction during respirations (blue), (a). Schematic ultrasound image showing to-and-fro movement along the pleural line during respirations. The two pleura are not distinctly visible with ultrasound and it is the presence of lung sliding (gray arrow heads) that indicates the pleura are together (b). A lines are visible in both images, although it may be easier to see lung sliding when A lines are not visible (see Fig. 8).

(Fig. 8; video 3.2). Lung sliding is easier to see when A lines are not visible and the angle of insonation is deferred from 90 degrees.

- Change the angle the ultrasound beam strikes the pleural line by placing the transducer over a single rib head referred to as the dead bat sign (also called the one-eyed gator; Fig. 9; video 3.3).
- Decrease the depth and frequency settings to make the pleural line larger and "grainier", which makes lung sliding easier to appreciate.
- Decrease the gain setting on the ultrasound machine to make the pleural line "grainier" (video 3.4).

Note: if the depth and gain settings are decreased to help identify lung sliding, they should be increased once lung sliding is assessed as low gain and depth settings may prevent other normal structures and lung surface artifact from being identified (e.g. the abdominal curtain sign, B lines, consolidations, etc.).

- Finally, turning off the various smoothing and artifact minimization filters, which are available on many ultrasound machines, will often make it easier to identify lung sliding.

QR
Video 3.2.
Insonation change.

QR
Video 3.3.
Dead bat.

QR
Video 3.4.
Gain change.

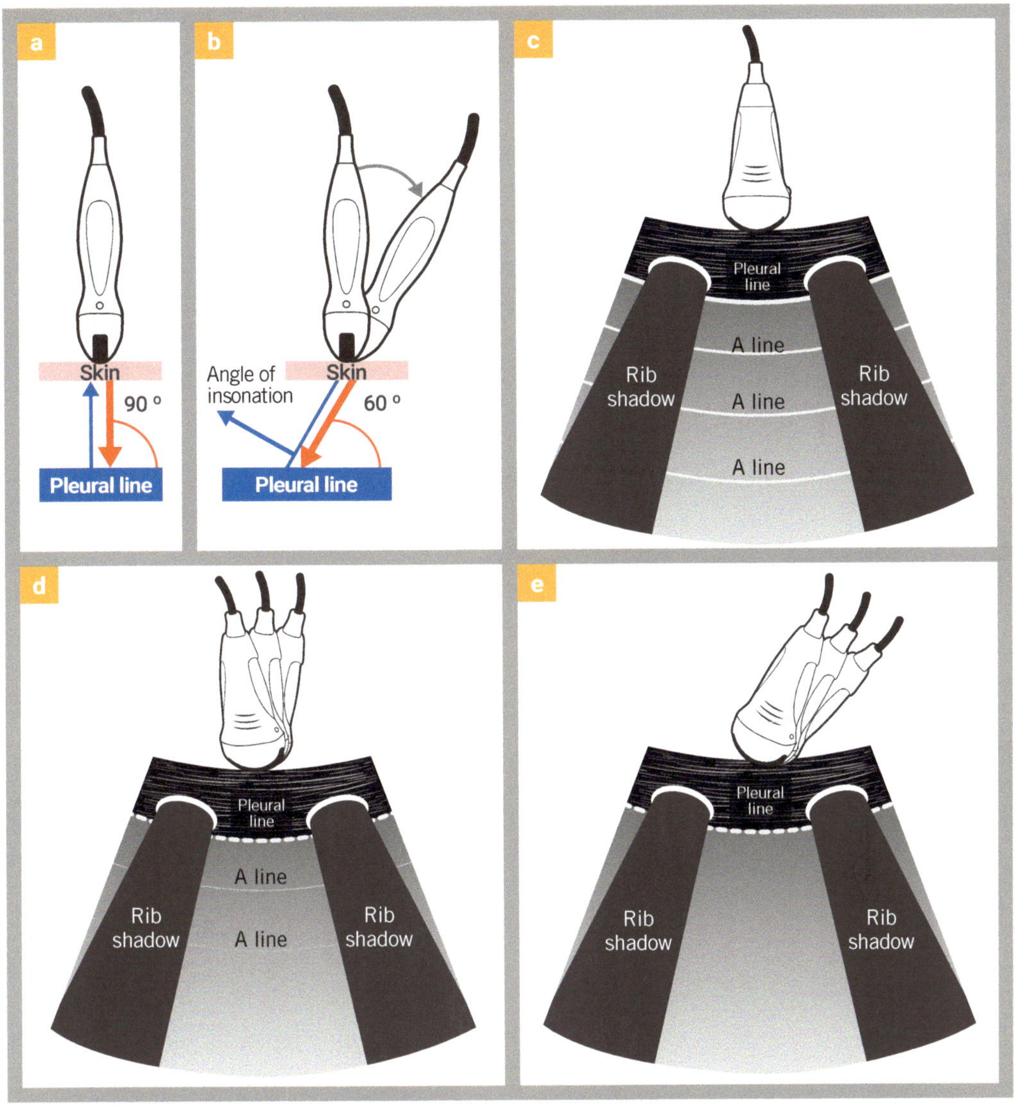

Figure 8. Schematic images depicting the angle of insonation the ultrasound beam (a and b), and schematic ultrasound image obtained with the transducer perpendicular, fanned or rocked relative to the pleural line (c and e). Schematic drawing of the transducer at 90 degrees to the pleural line; this creates two highly reflective surfaces parallel to each other (transducer surface and the pleural line) causing the ultrasound beam to be reflected back and forth between the two structures (a). Schematic drawing with the transducer fanned from a 90 degree angle; less of the ultrasound beam (thin blue arrow) is reflected back and forth between the transducer surface and the pleural line causing the pleural line to appear "grainier" and A lines to be less visible (b). Schematic ultrasound image of the transducer aligned perpendicular to the pleural line, which causes the pleural line to be brighter and maximizes visibility of A lines, but makes lung sliding more difficult to visualize (difficult lung sliding is depicted by a solid pleural line) (c). Schematic ultrasound image of the transducer after fanning 20 dregrees from 90, which changes the angle the ultrasound beam strikes the pleural line making it appear "grainier" (dotted pleural line), which also makes A lines less visible and lung sliding easier to identify (d). Continued fanning of the transducer to an angle at which A lines become invisible, which is often an angle at which the pleural line is easiest to assess for lung sliding (e).

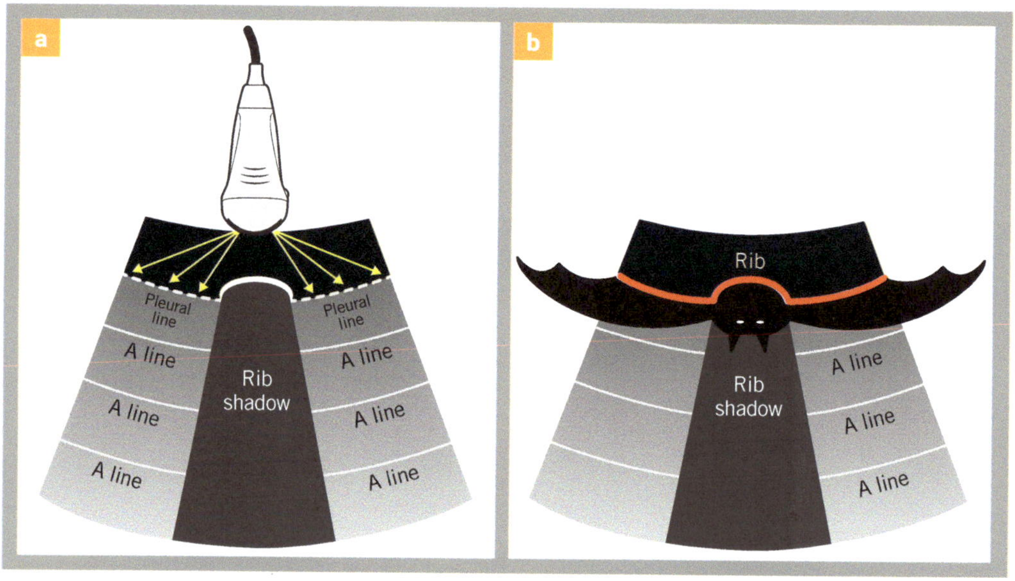

Figure 9. Schematic ultrasound images depicting the transducer centered over a single rib; changing the angle, the ultrasound beam strikes the pleural line, making it appear grainier and therefor easier to visualize lung sliding (dotted pleural line) (a). For orientation, placing the transducer over a single rib resembles an upside down or "dead bat" where structures are reversed to the normal bat sign; the body represents the proximal rib surface and the wings represent the pleural line (b).

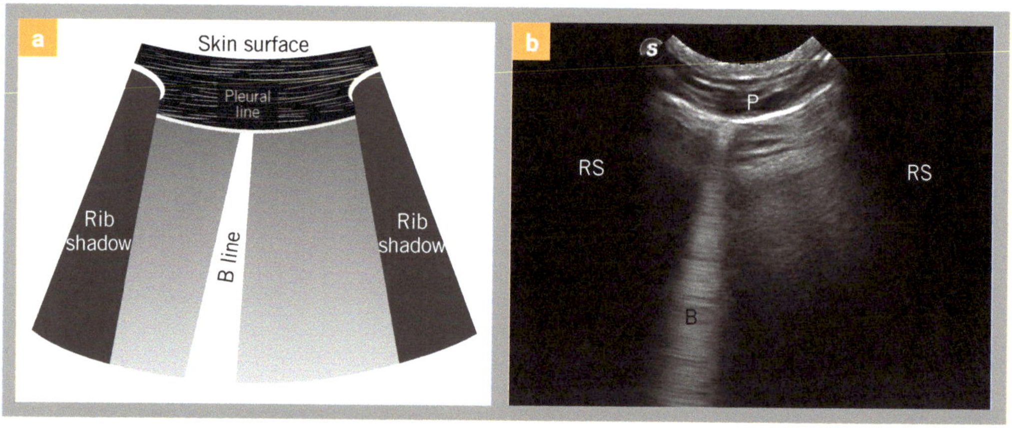

Figure 10. Schematic ultrasound image depicting a single B line (a), and its corresponding ultrasound still image (b) that was identified in a healthy dog. B lines appear as hyperechoic vertical lines that move to-and-fro with lung sliding, often extending to the far field of the image. B; B line, P; pleural line, RS; rib shadow.

B LINES

B lines, occasionally referred to as lung rockets, comet-tail artifacts and ring-down artifacts, are sonographic laser-like vertical hyperechoic projections that arise from the lung surface (Fig. 10; video 3.5). Based on recent consensus guidelines the term B line is the preferred standardized nomenclature[5].

B lines, which originate from the visceral pleura of the lung surface, will extend from the pleural line when the lung surface is in contact with the thoracic wall. Therefore, the identification of B lines originating at the pleural line rules out pneumothorax. As there are a number of artifacts that can be mistaken for B lines (e.g. Z lines, I lines, and E lines), strict criteria should be met to ensure the artifacts encountered are B lines.

QR
Video 3.5.
Multiple B lines.

B lines have been identified in up to 10 to 30 % of healthy dogs and cats, with a correlation of more B lines being identified as more lung surface area is evaluated[6-10]. They are visible when the transducer is placed over peripheral lung regions with an increased tissue-air ratio (see Chapter 6), and can occur in healthy animals because of interlobar septa or regions with micro atelectasis at the lung periphery. In healthy animals B lines are most often identified in isolation or in pairs (Fig. 11; video 3.6) within a single sonographic window.

B line criteria:

The following three criteria are always present with B lines:

- They are vertical white lines.
- They originate at the lung surface (i.e. at the pleural line of healthy animals if the two pleura are in contact).
- They move in synchrony with lung sliding, swinging to-and-fro with lung sliding during the respiratory cycle.

The following two criteria are usually, but not always present:

- They extend to the far field.
- They obscure A lines if present.

QR
Video 3.6.
Single B line.

The identification of 3 B lines in a single sonographic window is possible, but considered rare in heathy cats and dogs (Fig. 12)[9,10]. It is also possible to identify B lines at more than one sonographic window on either or both hemithoraces, depending on the number of lung regions scanned; however, finding even a low number of B lines (e.g. 1 or 2) in multiple lung windows (e.g. more than two sites on a hemithorax) should prompt consideration of lung pathology. In this setting, additional PLUS findings should be assessed to create the PLUS profile, which in combination with other clinical, history, and POCUS findings helps determine if pathology is truly

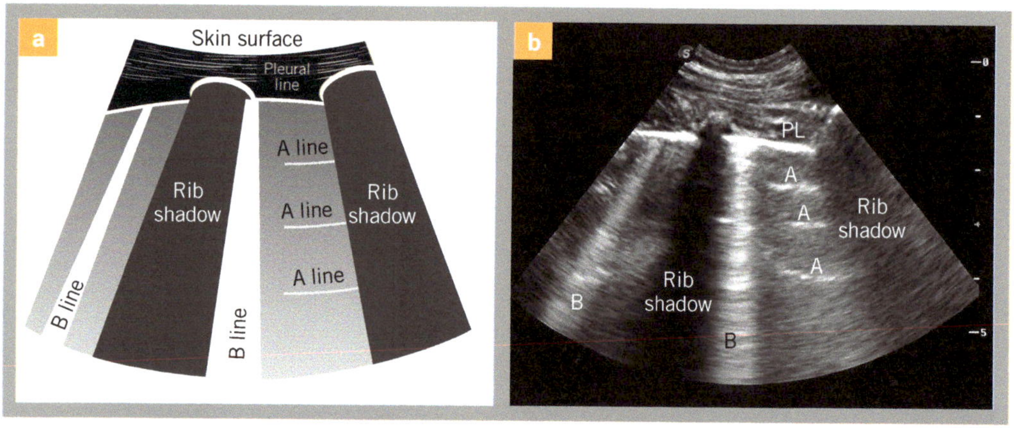

Figure 11. Schematic ultrasound image depicting 2 B lines (a), and its corresponding ultrasound still image that was identified in a healthy 4-year-old domestic short-haired cat (b). A lines are partially visible on the right side of the image where the ultrasound beam is striking the pleura at a more perpendicular angle. The pleural line is curving slightly away from the transducer in this image, which can be a normal variation, particularly in cats. Note that the width of B lines may vary slightly. B; B line, P; pleural line, RS; rib shadow.

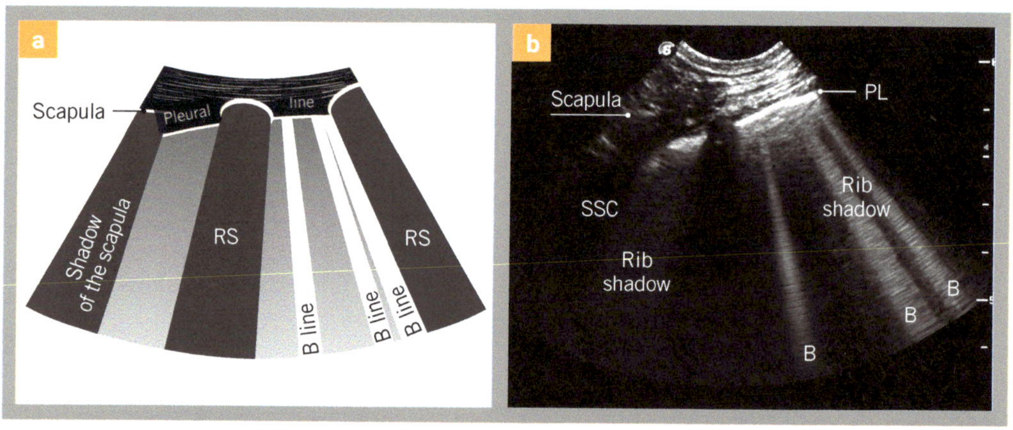

Figure 12. Schematic ultrasound image depicting 3 single B lines (a), and its corresponding still ultrasound image identified in a healthy 2-year-old small breed dog (b). Note that the soft tissue structures above the pleural line get thicker to the left of the image due to the presence of the flexor muscles of the shoulder being encountered (the transducer is close to the cranial border of the sonographically-defined thoracic borders). The surface of the scapula is also just visible on the left of the ultrasound images as a very short weakly hyperechoic horizontal line giving rise to the acoustic shadowing. B; B line, PL; pleural line, RS; rib shadow, SSC; bone shadow of the scapula.

present, and if so, narrow differential diagnosis (see Chapter 7). Identification of more than 3 B lines in a single sonographic window is indicative of lung pathology (see Chapter 6; video 3.5).

Changing the angle of insonation makes B lines more or less visible, depending on the angle at which the ultrasound beam interacts with the lung surface. In general, it is recommended to assess B lines when the angle between the ultrasound beam and the pleural line is 90 degrees, when A lines are most visible, and the pleural line is bright.

CURTAIN SIGNS

Normal curtain signs are created when air-filled lung overlies soft tissue structures within the thorax. The presence of air-filled lung overlying soft tissues creates a sharp vertical edge artifact demarcating the transition between lung (reverberation artifact) and the soft tissue structures they overly[1]. Think of the aerated lung border as acting like a "curtain"; when it fills with air and expands, it is drawn over other organs, momentarily obscuring them from view, like a curtain is drawn across a window obscuring what is visible through the window. The underlying organs disappear as the lung expands across them on inspiration and reappear as the lung contracts on exhalation. In healthy patients, depending on the area the transducer is placed on the thorax, different soft tissue structures can be seen partially covered by air-filled lung. As such, there are two main curtain signs normally identified:

- The abdominal curtain sign which can be seen when air-filled lung overlies the diaphragm and soft tissue structures of the abdomen at the costophrenic recess (video 3.7).
- The cardiac curtain sign which is seen when air-filled lung overlies the soft tissue structures of the heart at the cardiac notch (video 3.8).
- The abdominal curtain sign is the most evident and commonly assessed curtain sign and will be discussed in detail below.

QR
Video 3.7.
Abdominal curtain.

QR
Video 3.8.
Cardiac curtain.

Abnormal curtain signs can arise for several reasons. Because the sharp vertical edge artifact of a curtain sign is created by air overlying soft tissue structures, it is not restricted to air-filled lung, and can also be created when free air in the pleural space overlies soft tissue structures, referred to as abnormal pneumothorax-induced curtain signs (see Chapter 4). It is therefore important not to confuse the cyclical respiratory driven movement of a curtain sign for lung sliding, as curtain signs maybe seen when pneumothorax is present (absence of lung sliding) and when air-filled lung is present (presence of lung sliding) at the costophrenic recess.

Additionally, when pleural effusion is present curtain signs can also be created when air-filledlung overlies the pleural effusion, expanding and contracting across it, which is an abnormal pleural effusion induced curtain sign.

Abdominal curtain signs

In healthy animals, the abdominal curtain sign is the sonographically-defined caudal border of the lungs that can be seen when the transducer is positioned transthoracically, half over lung and half over visible abdomen (Fig. 13);

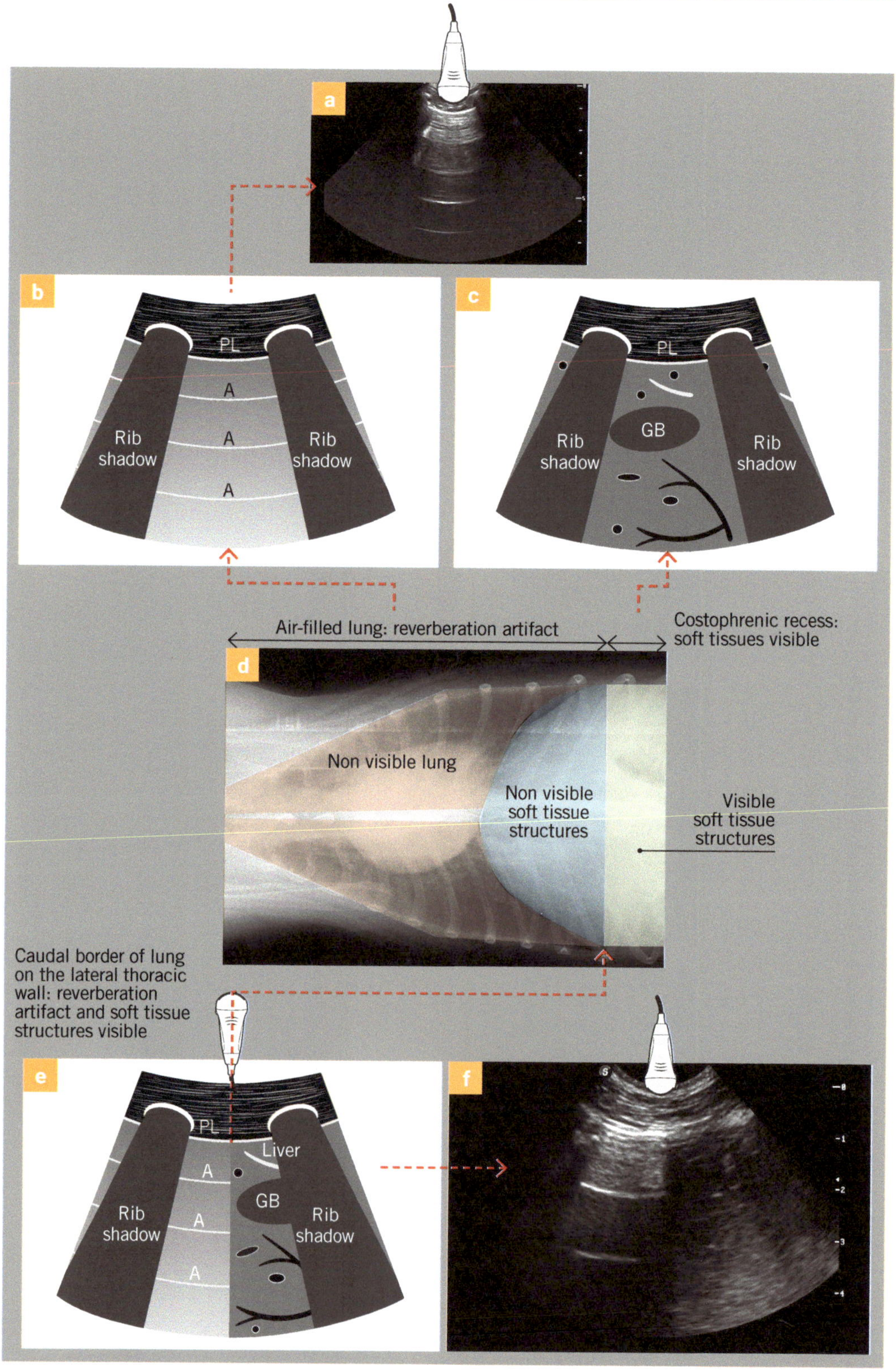
a
b
PL
A
A
A
Rib shadow
Rib shadow
c
PL
GB
Rib shadow
Rib shadow
Air-filled lung: reverberation artifact
Costophrenic recess: soft tissues visible
d
Non visible lung
Non visible soft tissue structures
Visible soft tissue structures
Caudal border of lung on the lateral thoracic wall: reverberation artifact and soft tissue structures visible
e
PL
Liver
A
A
A
GB
Rib shadow
Rib shadow
f

Figure 13. Ventral dorsal thorax radiograph demonstrating schematic ultrasound images obtained based on where the transducer is placed over the thorax. Upper still ultrasound image: the transducer is placed over lung (radiographically outlined in pink; the lung itself is not visible). The ultrasound beams are reflected from the soft tissue-to-air interface creating A lines (a). Upper middle left schematic ultrasound image demonstrating the classic bat sign (b). Upper middle right schematic ultrasound image; the transducer is placed over only soft tissue structures of the abdomen, caudal to the lungs (radiographically outlined in green) and the ultrasound beam is transmitted through the soft tissues allowing them to be identified on the ultrasound image (c). Lower middle still ultrasound image; on the left side of the ultrasound image the transducer is situated over lung, which reflects the ultrasound beam from the soft tissue-to-air interface, giving rise to A lines. On the right side of the ultrasound image the transducer is situated over soft tissue structures of the abdomen which transmits the ultrasound beam (green dotted arrow) allowing the underlying tissue to be visualized to the far field of the image (d). Lower bottom schematic ultrasound image: the transducer is centered over the caudal lateral border of the lung (identified by the dotted red arrow), the ultrasound beam being half over lung and half over soft tissue structures. Air within the lungs creates reverberation artifact in half the image (rendering the soft tissue structures deep to the lung nonvisible —radiographically blue shaded area). Where the ultrasound beam is not impeded by air it will pass through the soft tissue structures (radiographically shaded in green) causing the vertical sharp artifact at the transition from reverberation artifact to soft tissue structures referred to as the curtain sign. A; A line, P; pleural line, RS; rib shadow, GB; gallbladder.

air in the lung creates reverberation artifact that obliterates the superimposed soft tissue structures of the abdomen, while the ultrasound beam is transmitted through the soft tissue structures caudal to the lung (Fig. 13; video 3.7). This creates a sharp vertical artifact demarcating the transition between lung (reverberation artifact) and soft tissue structures visible through the costophrenic recess caudal to the lung (Fig. 14). The costophrenic recess is a part of the pleural space which allows the lung to expand caudally during inspiration, accounting for the caudal movement of the curtain sign on inspiration.

The appearance of abdominal structures will vary as the transducer (in perpendicular orientation to the ribs) is swept ventrally and dorsally along the abdominal curtain sign, and between the left and right sides of the thorax (e.g. the spleen and stomach wall [video 3.9] will comprise the abdominal structures on the left side of the patient while the liver is more visible on the right [video 3.7]). When larger solid tissue structures are visible (e.g. liver, spleen, kidneys), the curtain sign is easier to visualize, however, when only the gastrointestinal wall and luminal gas is visible (e.g. stomach wall or intestinal wall) on the soft tissue side of the curtain sign, it is easier to confuse the normal abdominal structures for lung pathology (Fig. 14; video 3.9). The abdominal curtain sign is also visible with the transducer oriented parallel to the ribs because of the shape of the most lateral caudal lung margins, which curve and get larger caudodorsally.

When created by air-filled lung of healthy patients, the abdominal curtain sign displays distinct characteristics; during inspiration, as the lung expands into the costophrenic recess the abdominal curtain sign appears to move caudally covering more of the intraabdominal structures (Fig. 15; video 3.7). However, the movement of the abdominal curtain is caused by lung expansion and therefore not perfectly synchronous to the movement of the intra-abdominal structures which occur because of diaphragmatic activity. As a result of these distinct features, there are several

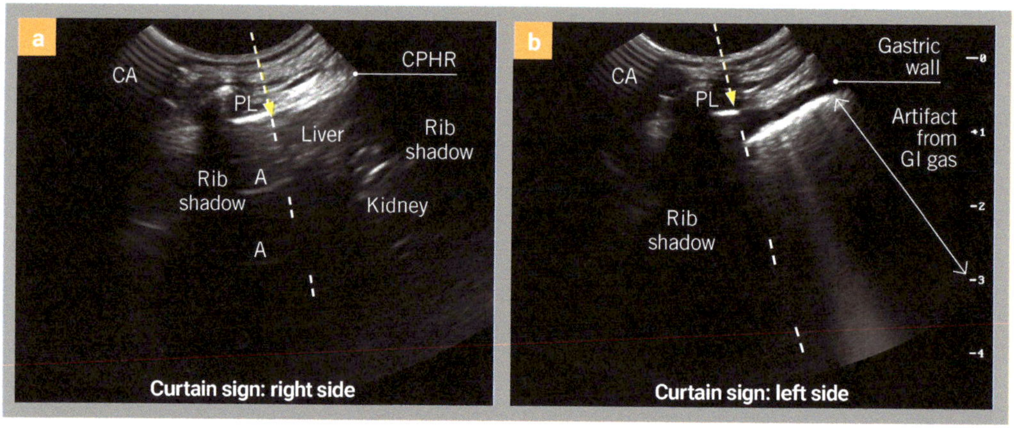

Figure 14. Ultrasound still images of the curtain sign identified in a healthy 2-year-old Labrador Retriever. (a) Curtain sign on the right side of the dog showing soft tissue structures (liver and kidney) throughout the image. The transition from reverberation artifact of the lung to visible soft tissue structures of the abdomen is easier to appreciate as there is a reverberation to soft tissue interface visible as a vertical line throughout the entire ultrasound image (a). Curtain sign on the left side of the dog placed over the stomach wall which contains gas. The only soft tissue visible caudal to the lung in this case is the wall of the stomach because there is intraluminal gas present below the stomach wall. This makes the curtain sign more difficult to identify as the reverberation artifact from the lung to soft tissue interface of the stomach wall is very thin. The reverberation artifact from lung to reverberation artifact of intestinal gas is difficult to differentiate, and it is easy to mistake GI artifact for lung artifact (e.g. ring down artifact in the GI tract can resembles B lines). Yellow dotted arrow represents the caudal border of the lung on the lateral thoracic wall. Broken dotted white line represents the curtain sign (transition of reverberation artifact of the lung visible abdominal structures). CA; contact artifact, PL; pleural line, RS; rib shadow, A; A lines, CPHR; costophrenic recess, GI; gastrointestinal.

QR

Video 3.9.
Left stomach curtain.
The movement of the curtain sign may be confused for lung sliding; both should be assessed carefully.

criteria that can be distinguished in healthy patients with a normal abdominal curtain sign: 1) there should only ever be one abdominal curtain sign visible at the caudal lung border; 2) which should always be visible throughout the entire respiratory cycle; and 3) although it may move slightly out of sync with the abdominal content and diaphragmatic activity, both the curtain sign and visible abdominal soft tissue structures should move in the same direction during the respiratory cycle. To avoid confusing rib shadows for the curtain sign, the curtain sign should be assessed when it is centred between two ribs, or located just caudal to the more cranial rib, at the end of expiration. Although the normal curtain sign may disappear as it passes under ribs (through rib shadows) or extends beyond the caudal border of the ultrasound image, it should not fade within the image itself (e.g. suddenly appear or disappear without moving out of the ultrasound image); it is always present in healthy animals.

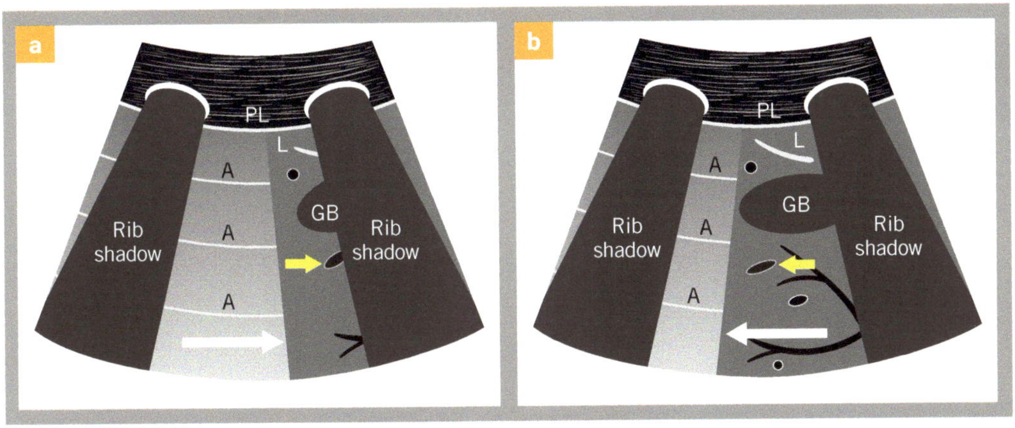

Figure 15. Schematic ultrasound images of the abdominal curtain sign with the transducer transverse to the ribs and the marker directed cranial. During inspiration the curtain sign (white arrow) and abdominal contents (yellow arrow) are shown sliding caudally in sync with each other (a). During expiration the curtain sign and abdominal contents are shown moving cranially together. The liver and gallbladder, hepatic and portal veins are shown (b). A; A lines, P; pleural line, L; liver, GB; gallbladder, RS; rib shadow.

Identification of the abdominal curtain sign:

- Allows operator to know where the externally placed transducer is located relative to the internal anatomy of the thorax. As the location of the caudal PLUS border, relative to intercostal spaces will vary depending upon species, breed, respiratory effort, underlying abdominal and thoracic pathology and patient position, it is extremely difficult to predict the sonographically-defined caudal PLUS border of dogs and cats using external landmarks.
- Allows subsequent identification of the most caudodorsal thoracic site where pleural air will accumulate in the sternal/standing patient, and the most caudal ventral border which is helpful in differentiating pleural and pericardial fluid as well as identifying smaller quantities of pleural effusion in the sternal/standing patient (see Chapter 2).
- Helps avoid the confusion of abdominal structures and extrathoracic pathology for lung and pleural space pathology (video 9).
- Allows several pathologies to be diagnosed when the curtain sign is no longer normal, including lung consolidation, pleural effusion and pneumothorax (see separate Chapters for details).

THE PERICARDIODIAPHRAGMATIC (PD) WINDOW

The PD window is defined when the transducer is positioned over the thorax and orientated perpendicular to the ribs such that both the heart (cranially) and diaphragm/abdominal contents (caudally) are visible within the same window. The PD window can be identified on both the left and right side of most dogs and cats, although its appearance varies depending if the heart is in contact with the diaphragm or if lung is superimposed over the two (Figs. 16 and 17).

Mediastinal triangle visible at the PD window

In healthy animals, the soft tissue-to-air interface created by lung being superimposed over abdominal soft tissues (the abdominal curtain sign) prevents the diaphragm from being visualized as it curves away from the thoracic wall. Therefore, on both the right and left sides of the thorax, the abdominal curtain sign always appears as a sharp vertical edge artifact extending through the far field of the image, with one exception, where the heart and diaphragm contact each other ventrally at the PD window (Fig. 16; video 3.10). A small triangle of tissue (fat) at the apex of the heart, referred to as the mediastinal triangle (MT), transmits ultrasound allowing the diaphragm to be visualized as it curves away from the thoracic wall. The heart's left ventricular free wall contacts the diaphragm and the mediastinal fat sits between the heart and diaphragm (Fig. 16c–d). If the diaphragm is seen curving away from the thoracic wall at any location other than the PD window, lung or pleural space pathology should be suspected[1] (see Chapters 5–7). Note: Do not confuse the mediastinal triangle for lung consolidation or other pathology. To find the PD window sweep ventrally and cranially along the abdominal curtain sign until the heart and diaphragm are visible in the same window (video 3.11).

QR
Video 3.10.
Curtain to PD window.

QR
Video 3.11.
Heart, lung, liver, PD.

Mediastinal triangle obscured by lung at the PD window

In many healthy cats and a few dogs the heart may not contact the diaphragm. In these cases, a region of aerated lung is visible between the heart and the diaphragm at the PD window, which allows both the cardiac curtain and abdominal curtain signs to be visualized in the same sonographic window as aerated lung overlies and obscures the mediastinal triangle (Fig. 17; video 3.12).

Identifying the PD window allows pleural and pericardial fluid to be easily differentiated (see Chapter 5).

QR
Video 3.12.
Lung superimposed over the heart and abdominal structures at PD window.

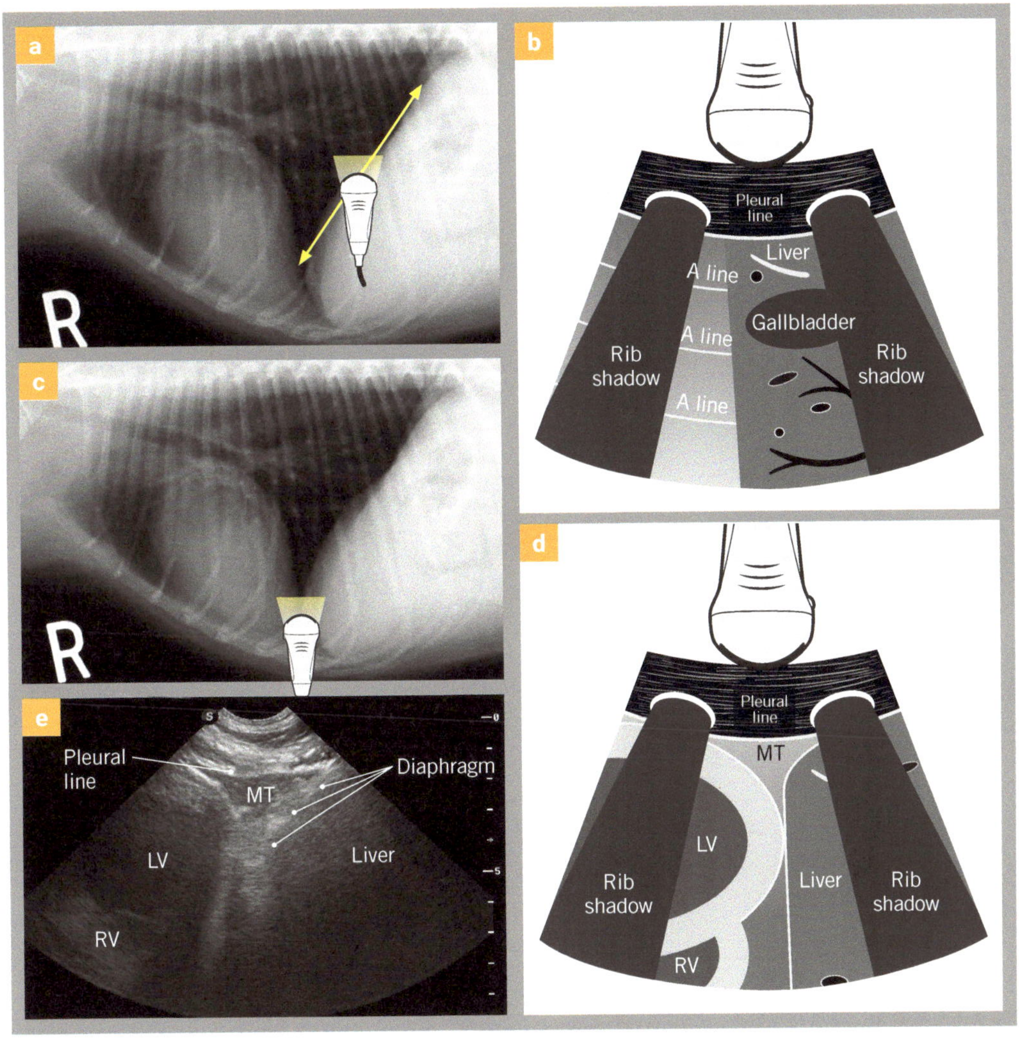

Figure 16. Radiograph, schematic ultrasound and still ultrasound images of a healthy dog. Radiograph of a dog showing the transducer positioned over the abdominal curtain sign (a). Schematic ultrasound image. Although the diaphragm is visible curving away from the thoracic wall on radiographs, when the transducer is placed over the abdominal curtain sign air within the lung prevents the diaphragm from being visualized once it curves away from the thoracic wall (b). Radiograph demonstrating positioning of the transducer, orientated transverse to the ribs, in order to visualize the heart and diaphragm in the same sonographic window, referred to as the pericardiodiaphragmatic (PD) window (c). Schematic ultrasound image demonstrating the apex of the heart in contact with the diaphragm including the mediastinal triangle (MT), which transmits ultrasound allowing the diaphragm to be visualized curving away from the thoracic wall (d). Ultrasound still image of (b) obtained from the left side of the thoracic in a healthy dog demonstrating the MT, which allows the diaphragm to be seen curving away from the thoracic wall (vertical curtain sign is absent) at the PD window (e).

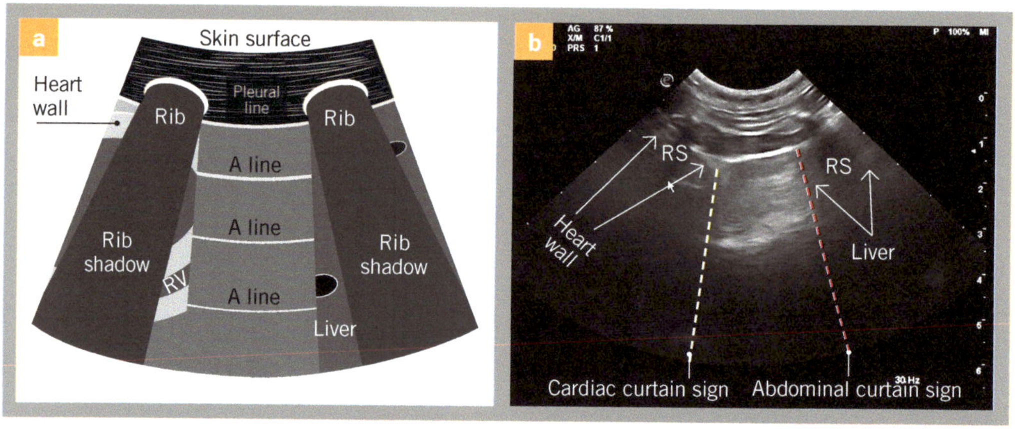

Figure 17. Schematic diagram (a) and ultrasound image (b) of the PD window with the transducer in perpendicular position to the ribs in a heathy cat or dog where the mediastinal triangle of fat is obscured by overlying aerated lung. At this window, when lung is superimposed over the heart and abdominal structures, the left ventricular free wall will not be seen contacting the diaphragm. In these cases the heart, pleural line and vertical edge artifact of the cardiac and abdominal curtain signs will be seen. RS; rib shadow, RV; right ventricle.

DRY LUNG

To conclude the lung surface is dry, specific binary questions are assessed at each sonographic window (e.g. dry lung at each window, yes/no), followed by the summation of all windows over each hemithorax and for the entire patient considering all clinical findings, which creates the PLUS profile (see Chapters 6 and 7). However, PLUS is a surface imaging technique and only reflects underlying lung pathology that reaches the lung surface. Fortunately most lung pathology appears to reach the lung surface and will be visible as either increased B lines or lung consolidation (see Chapters 6 and 7)[1,2]. The lung surface is considered dry at the specific sonographic window when the following two criteria are present:

1. The patient has lung sliding. As stated previously, lung sliding indicates the lung is in contact with the thoracic wall making it possible to assess if the lung surface is dry or lung pathology is present. The lung should not be assessed if it is not in contact with the thoracic wall (do not assess lung when lung sliding is absent; see Chapters 4–6).
2. There are 0 to 3 B lines in a single sonographic window. Up to 3 B lines in a single window can be considered normal in cats and dogs; however, as mentioned, the presence of any B line should be assessed considering the entire PLUS profile and complete clinical picture before concluding the lung is dry or underlying lung pathology is present at that specific transducer location (see Chapter 6).

Because PLUS scans multiple lung regions, the lung surface may appear dry in some areas but also contain lung pathology in others. It's also possible that each sonographic window may meet the criteria of dry lung, but the patient may still have lung pathology if multiple windows scanned contain one or

Detecting only A lines in the presence of lung sliding is indicative of dry lung at the transducer location, however, as A lines are not always visible (see A lines above), the authors prefer to define dry lung based on assessing lung sliding and determining the absence or number of B lines visible:

- Absence of B lines = dry lung at that transducer location.
- 3 or fewer B lines = dry lung at that transducer location.
- More than 3 B lines = lung pathology at that transducer location (Fig. 18; see Chapter 6).

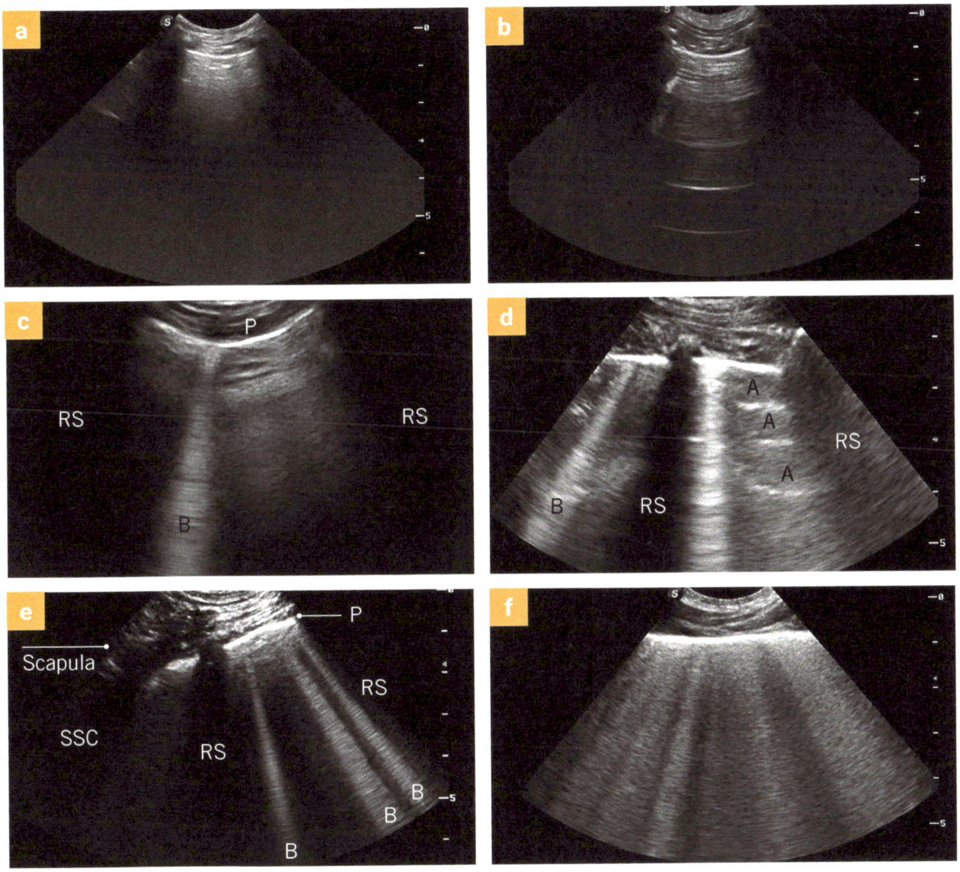

Figure 18. Ultrasound still images. No A lines or B lines visible (a). Only A lines and no B lines visible (b). Only a single B line visible (c). 2 B lines and A lines visible (d). 3 B lines and no A lines visible (e). In these five examples, there are ≤ 3 B lines, which meets the criteria for dry lung at that single sonographic window, irrespective of the presence or absence of A lines. More than 3 B lines visible (transducer is parallel to the ribs so there are no ribs or rib shadows visible) and an absence of A lines, indicating lung pathology is present (f). Lung sliding was not possible to demonstrate in a still image but was present at the transducer location in all six cases. Although the first 5 cases meet the definition of dry lung a teach specific sonographic window, the entire PLUS profile and all clinical findings must be assessed to determine if the lung are truly dry or contain underlying lung pathology (see Chapters 6 and 7). P; pleural line, A; A lines, B; B lines, RS; Rib shadow, SSC; shadow of the scapula.

more B lines. This emphasises the importance of considering the entire PLUS profile and all clinical findings to make a conclusion.

"SKI JUMP" SIGN

The "ski jump" sign is a newer sonographic finding that is used to describe the normal appearance of the sonographically-defined ventral thoracic border. When the transducer is orientated parallel to the ribs at the sonographically-defined ventral thoracic border (with the transducer marker directed dorsally), either lung or heart can be seen curving away from the transducer along the pectoral sternal muscles. This creates an ultrasound image with a similar appearance to an "Olympic ski jump" (Fig. 19; videos 3.13 and 3.14). The "ski jump" sign occurs where the parietal lining of the chest wall transitions onto the sternal muscles ventrally, and is comprised of either sternal/pectoral muscles interfacing with lung or sternal/pectoral muscles interfacing with cardiac muscle depending where along the thorax the transducer is situated (Fig. 19). The "ski jump" sign is used to rule out smaller volumes of pleural effusion that might otherwise be missed with the transducer orientated transverse to the ribs at the level of the costochondral junction (see Chapter 5).

QR
Video 3.13.
Ski jump lung.

LUNG PULSE

The lung pulse is the rhythmic to-and-fro, small beat to beat, oscillation of the pleura resulting from the radiation of the cardiac beat to the lung surface. In essence, the lung pulse is equivalent to a "mini lung slide", which occurs independent of the respiratory cycle, and indicates that the parietal and visceral pleura are in contact (video 3.15).

The presence of lung pulse rules out pneumothorax at the transducer location.

The limitation of the lung pulse is that it is more difficult to identify at lung regions more distal from the heart, and it is not present in well aerated lung where lung sliding becomes dominant and the lung is resistant to cardiac vibrations. The lung pulse has a significant role in diagnosis of single lung lobe intubation as lung sliding is absent over the nonintubated lung due to lack of air flow through the airways, but the lung pulse is still visible.

QR
Video 3.14.
Ski jump heart.

QR
Video 3.15.
Lung pulse.

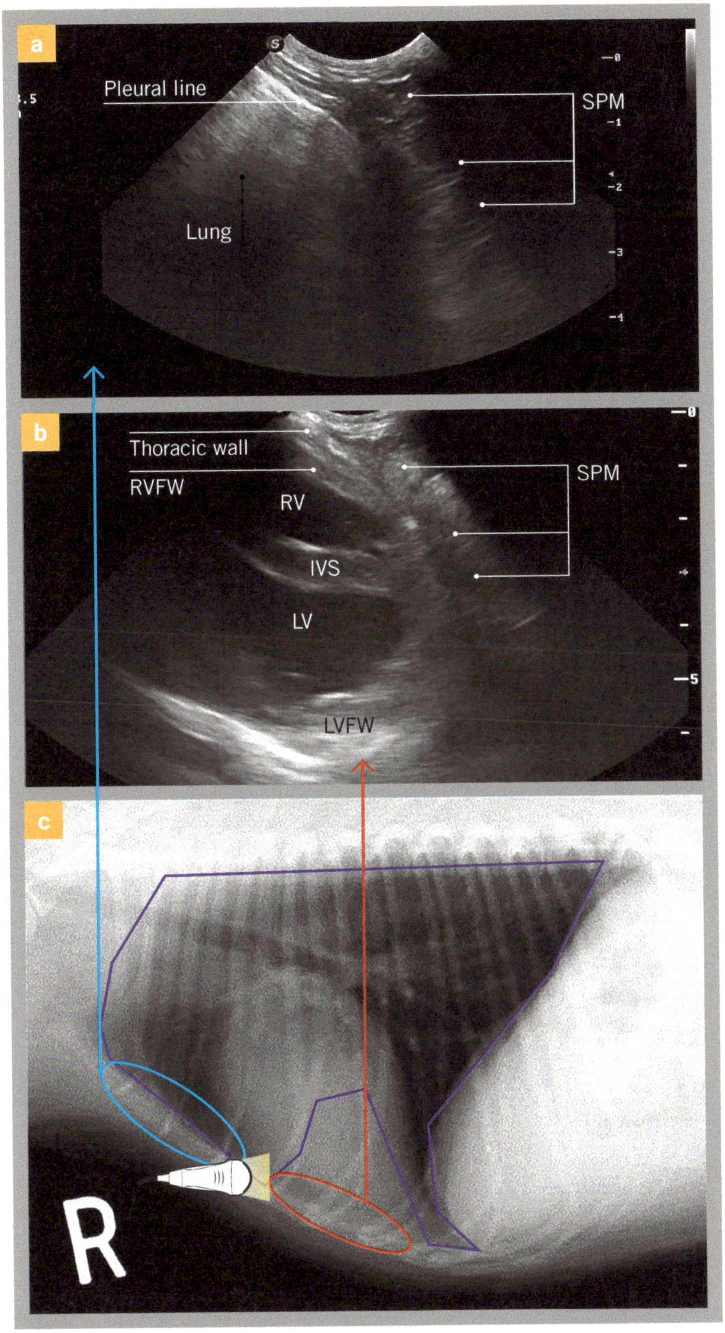

Figure 19. The "ski jump" sign. Ultrasound still images depicting the pleural line, sternal muscles and lung with the transducer orientated parallel to the ribs in the ventral pleural region (a). Ultrasound still image depicting the interface between the heart and sternal/pectoral muscles with the transducer orientated parallel to the ribs at the most ventral regions (b). Radiograph demonstrating parallel transducer orientation over lung (blue circle) and the heart (red circle) which gives rise to still ultrasound images a and b, respectively (c). LV; left ventricle, RV; right ventricle, IVS; interventricular septum; RVFW; right ventricular free wall, LVFW; left ventricular free wall, SPM; sternal pectoral muscles.

Z LINES, I LINES AND E LINES

Z lines, which are present in most healthy small animals[5], are a vertical, hyperechoic type of artifact that must be distinguished from B lines; Z lines have no known clinical significance (Z for zero significance), while B lines, as discussed, can exclude pneumothorax and/or define the presence of lung pathology (see Chapter 6). Although Z lines arise from the pleural line, they do not move with lung sliding because they do not originate at the lung surface; they have an extrapulmonary origin (proximal or distal to the pleural line), and typically appear as static vertical artifacts (the may move with contraction of the thoracic wall but do not move in sync with lung sliding). They do not erase A lines, they are ill-defined and they disappear after 2–5 cm (Figs. 20 and 21; video 3.16).

QR
Video 3.16.
Z lines.

I lines are short vertical reverberation artifacts, arising from the pleural line, moving in sync with lung sliding, but fade with increasing depth (Figs. 20 and 21; video 3.17). The clinical significance of I lines is unknown, often being identified in healthy animals[5]. It has been speculated that I lines may represent incomplete B lines (I for incomplete). In essence, they strongly resemble B lines, except they are shorter, less sonographically-visible, and do not define lung pathology. I lines are more readily identified with high-frequency linear transducers, which may be helpful, as the presence of I lines confirms the two pleura are in contact (like B lines they rule out pneumothorax).

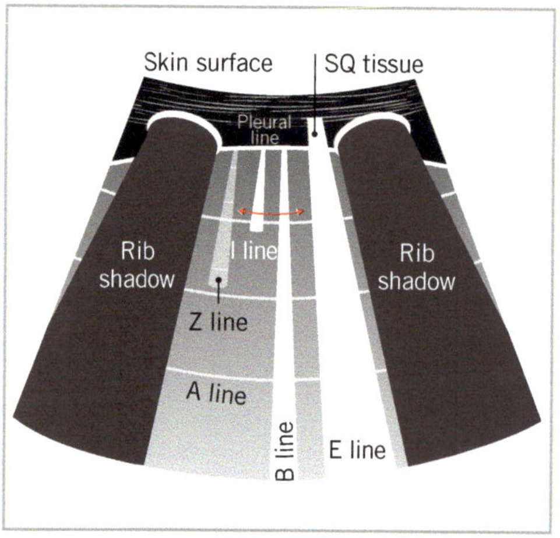

Figure 20. Schematic ultrasound image depicting the different lines that can be encountered during lung ultrasound. The red arrow indicates movement of the I line and B line with lung sliding. Z lines, E lines and A lines do not move with lung sliding.

QR
Video 3.17.
I line.

E lines are not present in healthy animals, although they are worth mentioning to avoid confusing them for B lines and/or I lines. E lines are the result of subcutaneous emphysema and the accumulation air within the subcutaneous tissues (Figs. 20 and 21; video 3.18). They can appear as comet-tail artifacts similar to B lines, however, they originate proximal to the pleural line (within the subcutaneous tissues), passing through and obliterating the pleural line (obscure the pleural line). They do not move in sync with lung sliding (they may move with thoracic wall contraction but remain independent of lung sliding) and may or may not extend to the far field of the ultrasound image. They can impede interpretation of the pleural line and other artifacts. It is sometimes possible to displace subcutaneous air by gently applying continual pressure to the ultrasound transducer (provided the patient is not too painful from concurrent injury to preclude persistent gentle pressure being applied), to allow the pleural line to be visualized.

SUMMARY

To be able to interpret PLUS pathology, it is essential to identify sonographic findings in normal animals; the six key "lines and signs" as well as identifying the pericardiodiaphragmatic window, defining dry lung, identifying the "ski jump" sign, the lung pulse, Z lines, I lines, and the five sonographically-defined pleural space and lung borders will make it easier to interpret abnormal findings and decrease the chances of false positive and false negative results.

QR
Video 3.18.
SQ emphysema.

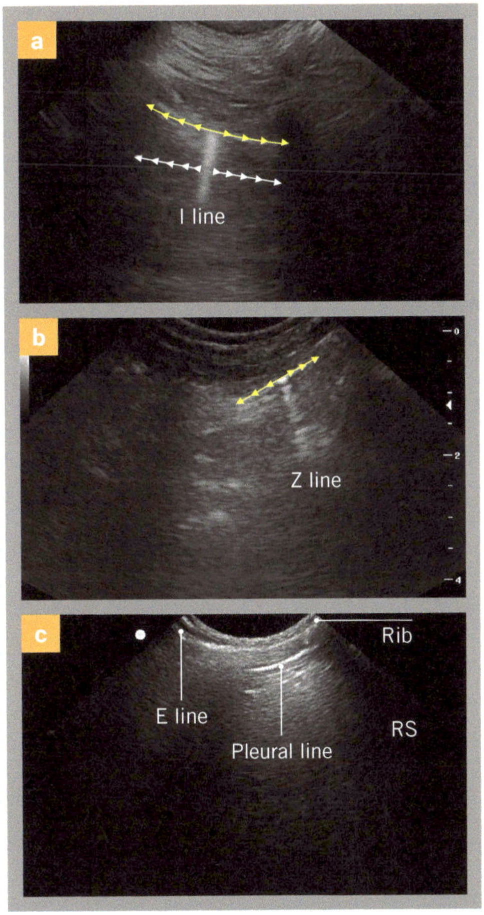

Figure 21. Ultrasound still images of I, Z and E lines. An I line is shown, which closely resembles a B line in that it originates at the pleural line (depicted in yellow) and moves to-and-fro (white arrow and arrow heads) with lung sliding (represented by yellow arrow heads) (a). A Z line is present which arises from the pleural line but remains static, not moving to-and-fro with lung sliding. Both I and Z lines fade after a short distance, although Z lines tend to be less distinct than I lines and where I lines tend to obliterate A lines when present, Z lines tend to accentuate the presence of A lines (b). E lines arise from the presence of air trapped in the subcutaneous tissues. They create comet-tail artifact that can be confused for B lines, although E lines are static, originate proximal to, and obliterate the pleural line (c). They obscure other clinically relevant lung and pleural space artifact. RS; rib shadow.

REFERENCES

1. Lee FC. Lung ultrasound-a primary survey of the acutely dyspneic patient. *J Intensive Care*, 2016, 4(1):57.
2. Lichtenstein D. Lung ultrasound in the critically ill. *Curr Opin Crit Care*, 2014, 20(3):315–322.
3. Kirkpatrick AW, Sirois M, Laupland KB, et al. Hand-held thoracic sonography for detecting post-traumatic pneumothoraces: the Extended Focused Assessment with Sonography for Trauma (EFAST). *J Trauma*, 2004, 57(2):288–295.
4. Martinez AN, Quinn C, Mihm F, Hennesse E. 1127: Lung Ultrasound: The fine line between diagnosing and ruling out pneumothorax. *Crit Care Med*, 2018, 46(1):547.
5. Volpicelli G, Elbarbary M, Blaivas M, et al. International evidence based recommendations for point-of-care lung ultrasound. *Intensive Care Med*, 2012, 38:577–591.
6. Martins A, Gouveia D, Cardoso A, et al. Incidence of Z, I and B lines detected with point of care ultrasound in healthy shelter dogs. *J Vet Emerg Crit Care*, 2019, 29:S17–S39.
7. Rademacher N, Pariaut R, Pate J, et al. Transthoracic lung ultrasound in normal dogs and dogs with cardiogenic pulmonary edema: a pilot study. *Vet Radiol Ultrasound*, 2014, 55(4):447–452.
8. Vezzosi T, Mannucci T, Pistoresi A, et al. Assessment of Lung Ultrasound B-Lines in Dogs with Different Stages of Chronic Valvular Heart Disease. *J Vet Intern Med*, 2017, 31(3):700–704.
9. Lisciandro GR, Fulton RM, Fosgate GT, Mann KA. Frequency and number of B-lines using a regionally based lung ultrasound examination in cats with radiographically normal lungs compared to cats with left-sided congestive heart failure. *J Vet Emerg Crit Care (San Antonio)*, 2017, 27(5):499-505.
10. Lisciandro GR, Fosgate GT, Fulton RM. Frequency and number of ultrasound lung rockets (B-lines) using a regionally based lung ultrasound examination named vet BLUE (veterinary bedside lung ultrasound exam) in dogs with radiographically normal lung findings. *Vet Radiol Ultrasound*, 2014 55(3):315–322.
11. Goffi A, Kruisselbrink R, Volpicelli G. The sound of air: point-of-care lung ultrasound in perioperative medicine. *Can J Anaesth*, 2018, 65(4):399–416.

04

CLINICAL APPLICATIONS OF PLUS: IS THERE PNEUMOTHORAX, YES/NO?

INTRODUCTION

The accuracy of ultrasound to identify pneumothorax in small animals varies from poor to excellent[1-4]. Although it is considered one of the most challenging diagnoses to make, the sonographic accuracy to diagnose pneumothorax can be improved with training, understanding of PLUS borders and abnormal curtain signs, and experience[1].

When the visceral pleura is separated from the parietal pleura by air, the visceral pleura becomes sonographically impossible to visualize as air does not transmit ultrasound. In this setting, the pleural line is still seen as a bright white line but it is only composed of the parietal pleura; lung sliding is lost because the visceral pleura of the lung no longer slides across the thoracic wall (video 4.1; see Chapter 3).

However, a soft tissue-to-air interface is still present with pneumothorax, comprised of the soft tissue structures of the thoracic wall to the level of the parietal pleura and the air within the pleural space, meaning reverberation artifact in the form of A lines will still be visible below the pleural line (Fig. 1). The lung will have some degree of atelectasis due to the presence of pneumothorax; however, this will not be sonographically detectable due to the presence of air between the lung surface and the parietal pleura.

QR
Video 4.1.
Lung sliding.

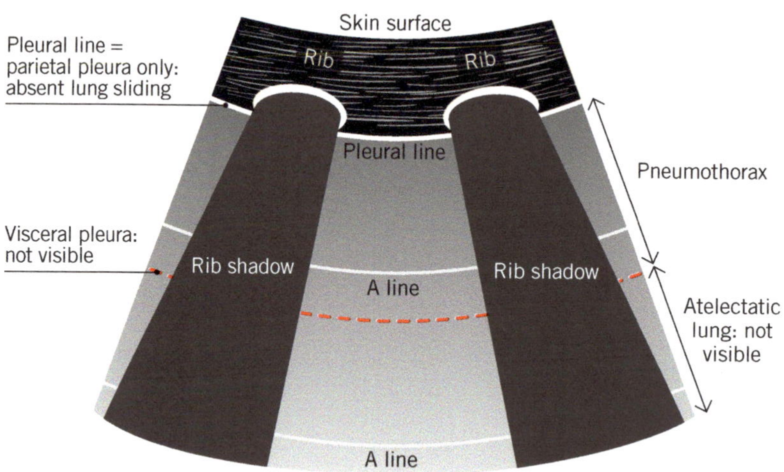

Figure 1. Schematic ultrasound image showing separation of the visceral pleura from the parietal pleura due to the presence of air in the pleural space (pneumothorax). In this instance, the pleural line (solid white line) is composed of only the parietal pleura and therefore lung sliding is absent (i.e. the two pleura are not in contact). The dotted red line represents the location of visceral pleura which is separated from the parietal pleura by air.

Key concepts

There are several essential concepts to understand when trying to sonographically identify pneumothorax:

- Air in the pleural space separates the visceral pleura from the parietal pleura, altering sonographic findings and creating pathognomonic signs of pneumothorax.
- Pneumothorax can only be ruled in or out at the location where the transducer is placed.
- Air is an enemy of ultrasound; with pneumothorax, the visceral pleura and lung surface cannot be visualized.
- Air rises to gravity independent sites (highest point) which varies with patient positioning.
- It is essential to assess the most sensitive sites for pneumothorax to avoid missing the diagnosis.

CRITERIA TO DIAGNOSE PNEUMOTHORAX

Evaluating patients for pneumothorax involves assessment of sonographic findings that rule out pneumothorax as well as sonographic findings that confirm its presence.

Pneumothorax should be suspected in the absence of rule out findings but can only be confirmed when rule in findings are present.

However, when the patient is in obvious respiratory distress, there is an absence of lung sliding, and the history and clinical findings are supportive of pneumothorax (e.g. absence of breath sounds in a trauma patient), thoracocentesis is immediately indicated.

Criteria to rule out pneumothorax

Pneumothorax can be ruled out at a specific transducer location when there is sonographic evidence that the visceral and parietal pleura are in contact. There are three sonographic findings that confirm the pleura are in contact; failure to identify these three findings does not confirm a diagnosis of pneumothorax.

The presence of complete lung sliding

The presence of complete lung sliding along the entire pleural line is specific and confirms that both pleura are in contact; it confidently rules out pneumothorax at the transducer location (video 4.2). However, complete lung sliding must be differentiated from the lung point, which appears as partial or intermittent lung sliding, and confirms pneumothorax (see below). Furthermore, lung sliding should not be presumed based on identification of the to-and-fro movement of an abdominal curtain sign as curtain sign movement can occur in the presence or absence of pneumothorax (see abnormal curtain signs below).

QR

Video 4.2.
No slide pneumotorax.

The absence of lung sliding is insufficient to diagnose pneumothorax.

Sometimes the shimmer of lung sliding is only visible along a section of the pleural line despite the pleura being in contact (video 4.3). This likely occurs because the ultrasound beam does not strike the pleural line at the same angle along its length. Changing the angle of the transducer and moving the transducer along the pleural line may make normal lung sliding easier to see (see Chapter 3).

QR
Video 4.3.
Difficult sliding.

The presence of B lines

B lines originating from the pleura rule out pneumothorax at that transducer location (see Chapter 3). When B lines are diffusely present due to underlying lung pathology (see Chapter 6), it is easy to exclude pneumothorax as a cause of dyspnea (video 4.4). However, given B lines are only present in up to 30% of healthy companion animals and at random locations along the lung surface, the absence of B lines, particularly at the caudodorsal site, does not confirm the diagnosis of pneumothorax. I lines also rule out pneumothorax at the transducer location (see Chapter 3). Finally, lung consolidation arising from the pleural line rules out pneumothorax at that transducer location (see Chapter 7).

QR
Video 4.4.
Multiple B lines.

Z lines are often confused for B lines but given Z lines are present in healthy animals and can be seen in cases with pneumothorax (See Chapter 3), they are not helpful at ruling out or confirming a diagnosis.

The presence of a lung pulse

The lung pulse is essentially a "mini lung slide" resulting from the oscillations of the heartbeat reaching the lung surface. The lung pulse rules out pneumothorax at sites it can be identified, which is often limited to lung regions in proximity to the heart (see video 3.15 in Chapter 3).

Criteria to rule in pneumothorax

The absence of lung sliding, B lines/lung consolidation, and a lung pulse, along with supportive history and clinical signs, should raise suspicion of pneumothorax; however, there are two key sonographic criteria that definitively confirm its presence.

The lung point

In a patient with pneumothorax, the lung point can be defined as the site within the thorax where the visceral pleura of the lung recontacts the parietal pleura of the thoracic wall. The lung point typically moves caudodorsally when the patient inspires and the lung expands (Fig. 2).

The lung point is considered pathognomonic for pneumothorax.

The lung point can appear differently depending on where and how the lung recontacts the thoracic wall within the ultrasound image, and if the underlying lung is dry or contains sonographically visible lung pathology. The lung may expand such that lung sliding is seen entering the ultrasound image from one side, advancing and retreating with the respiratory cycle. This creates a sonographic to-and-fro lung point (Fig 3; video 4.5). The to-and-fro lung point occurs when the lung is in contact with the thoracic wall below a region of pneumothorax; as the lung expands during inspiration, it slides along the thoracic wall into the region of pneumothorax.

QR
Video 4.5.
Dry lung point to-and-fro.

The lung may expand such that lung sliding suddenly appears within the center of the image enlarging and shrinking from a central point (Fig. 4) with the respiratory cycle, creating a central divergent (bidirectional) lung point (video 4.6). The divergent lung point occurs when the point of contact between lung surface and thoracic wall occurs within the central area of the ultrasound window; during inspiration the lung expands outward towards the thoracic wall until it suddenly appears within the central region of the sonographic window where pneumothorax was previously seen, radiating outwards from the central point of contact.

When the underlying lung contains pathology the lung point will contain B lines or consolidations (Fig. 5; videos 4.6 and 4.7). B lines, when they are present in conjunction with a complete lung slide, rule out pneumothorax (see Chapter 2); however, when they are present with a lung point, they definitively confirm the presence of a pneumothorax.

QR
Video 4.6.
Divergent B lung point.

QR
Video 4.7.
Lung point B line to-and-fro.

The sonographer has to carefully assess if the presence of B lines rule out pneumothorax when seen with complete lung sliding, or confirm its presence when seen with the lung point.

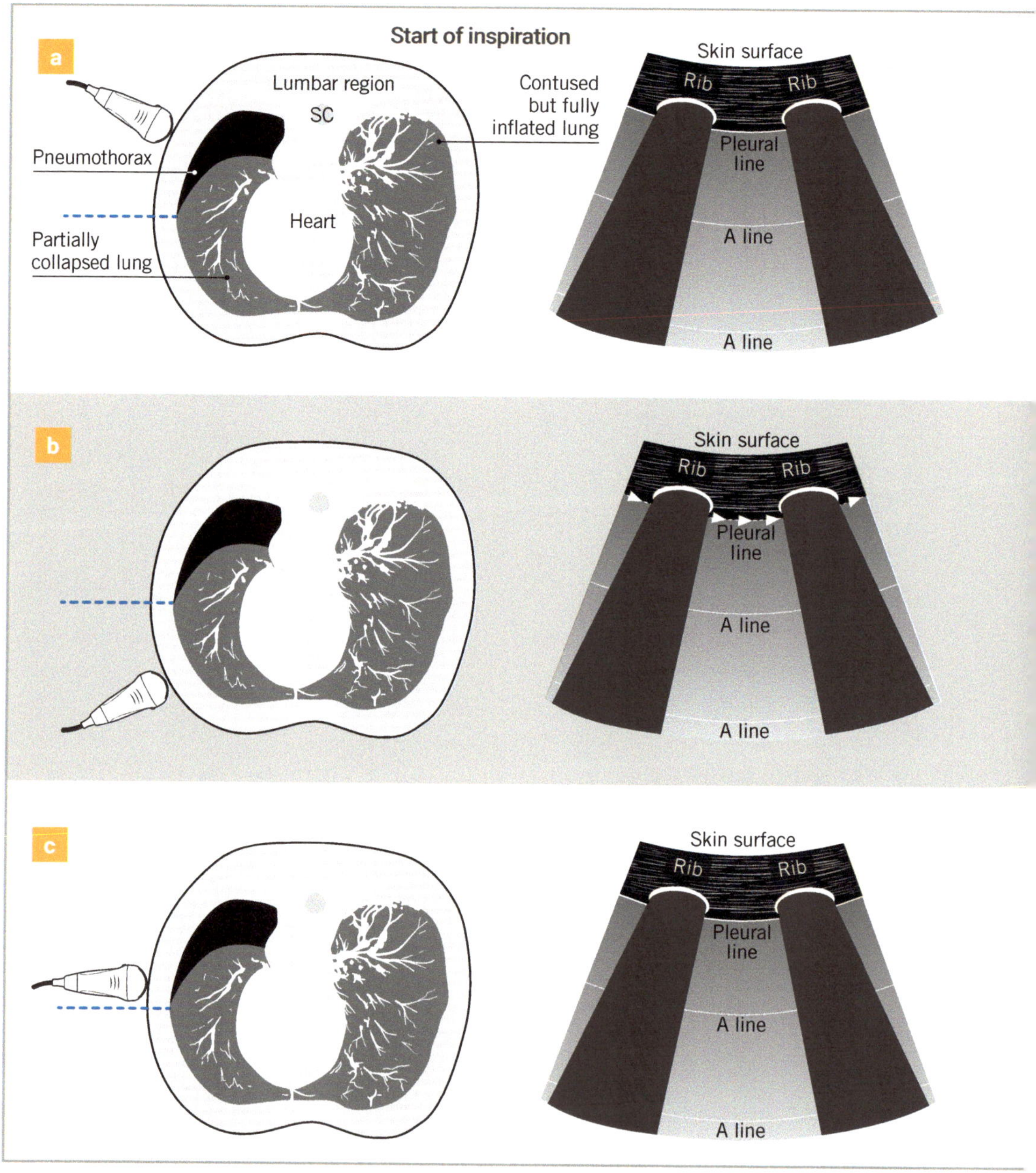

Figure 2. Ultrasound schematic images and computed tomography (CT) images of a patient in sternal recumbency. The blue dotted line identifies the contact point of the lung with the thoracic wall at end expiration and the red dotted arrow the point of lung contact with the thoracic wall at end inspiration. CT images are shown in transverse axis depicting transducer placement and how to find the lung point. The transducer is placed over an area of pneumothorax throughout the respiratory cycle and lung sliding is absent. The solid white line shown on the ultrasound schematic images represents the pleural line when there is an absence of lung sliding throughout the respiratory cycle (a). The transducer is placed over lung throughout the entire respiratory cycle and a complete lung sliding is present. The white dotted pleural line with arrow heads on the ultrasound

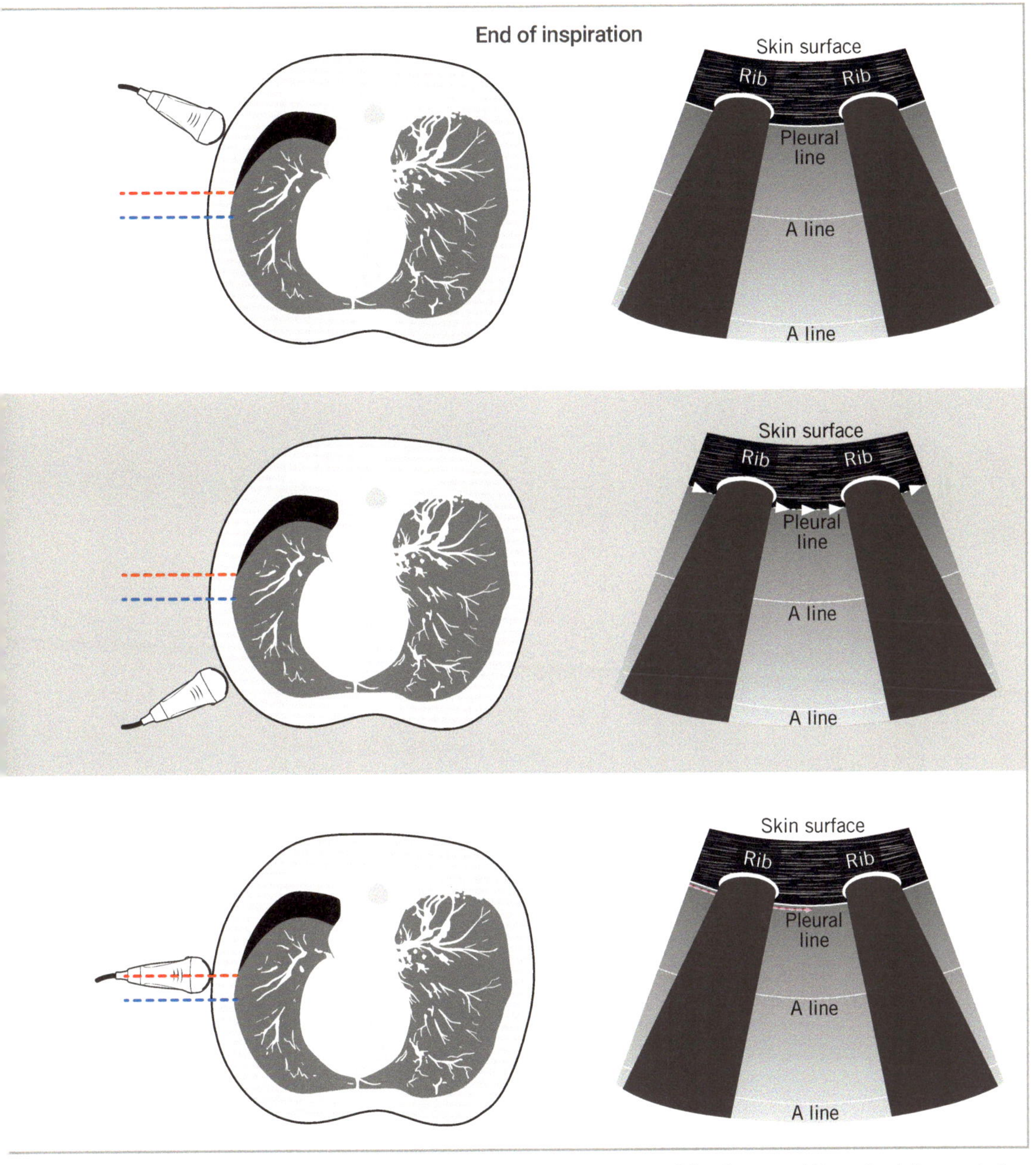

schematic images represents the pleural line when complete lung sliding is present throughout the respiratory cycle (b). The transducer is placed over the site just above the location where the lung recontacts the thoracic wall. Lung sliding is absent at the start of inspiration. The solid white line shown on ultrasound schematic images represents absence of lung sliding at the start of the inspiratory process. When the patient inspires the lungs expand and slide into the ultrasound window during the inspiratory phase; this is the lung point. The solid white line in the ultrasound schematic represents the absence of lung sliding in part of the image, while the pink dotted arrow represents lung sliding into the image from the left, creating a partial lung slide (see below). The blue dotted line identifies the contact point of the lung with the thoracic wall at end expiration and the red dotted arrow the point of lung contact with the thoracic wall at end inspiration (c).

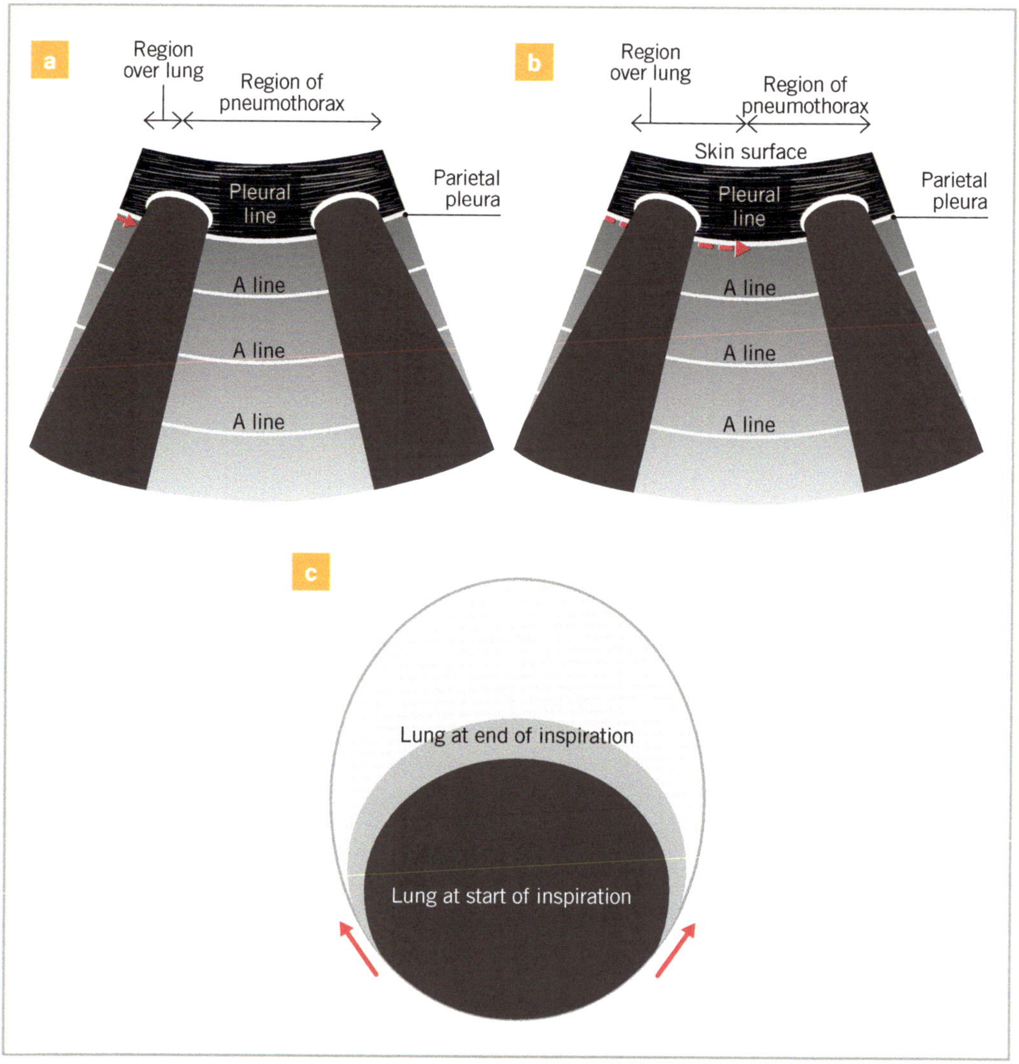

Figure 3. Ultrasound schematic images demonstrating a to-and-fro lung point. At the start of inspiration, the transducer is predominantly over a region of pneumothorax, with only a small portion of the transducer over a section of lung in contact with the thoracic wall at the very left side of the image (short red arrow) (a). During inspiration the lung will expand, sliding across the ultrasound image from left to right creating partial lung sliding. At the end of inspiration, the lung has reached its maximum expansion (long dotted red arrow), and begins to decrease in size during expiration (b). This will cause the lung to retreat to the size depicted in image a. Schematic representation of the lung expanding to create the to-and-fro lung point (c). The red arrow represents the lung sliding along the thoracic wall during inspiration, creating a to-and-fro lung point.

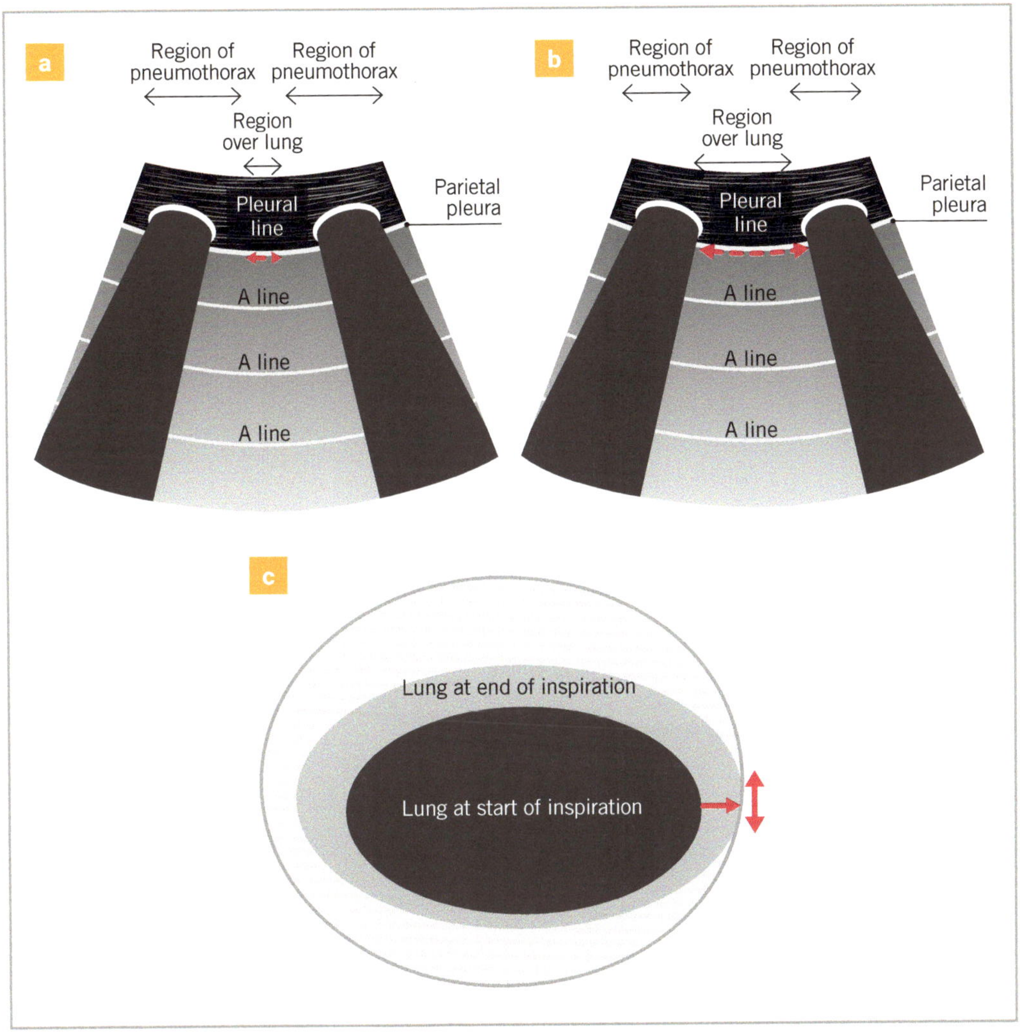

Figure 4. Ultrasound schematic images demonstrating a divergent (bidirectional lung point). At the start of inspiration, the transducer is predominantly over a region of pneumothorax, with only a small portion of the transducer over a section of lung in contact with the thoracic wall (short double headed red arrow). In this example a small section of lung is touching the thoracic wall in the centre of the image with free pleural air (pneumothorax) on either side of the lung point. During inspiration the lung will expand in both directions from the central point of contact, sliding in both directions, creating a divergent (bidirectional) partial lung slide (a). At the end of inspiration, the lung has reached its maximum expansion (long dotted double headed red arrow), and begins to decrease in size during expiration. This will cause the lung to retreat to the size depicted in image a. Lung sliding expands and decreases from a central point of contact with inspiration and expiration respectively, creating a divergent lung point (b). Schematic representation of the lung expanding to create the divergent lung point; dark grey circle represents the lung at the start of inspiration, and the light grey circle represent the lung at end expiration. The red arrows represent the lung expanding outward to contact the thoracic wall at a central location, and then sliding in either direction from the point of contact, creating a divergent lung point (c).

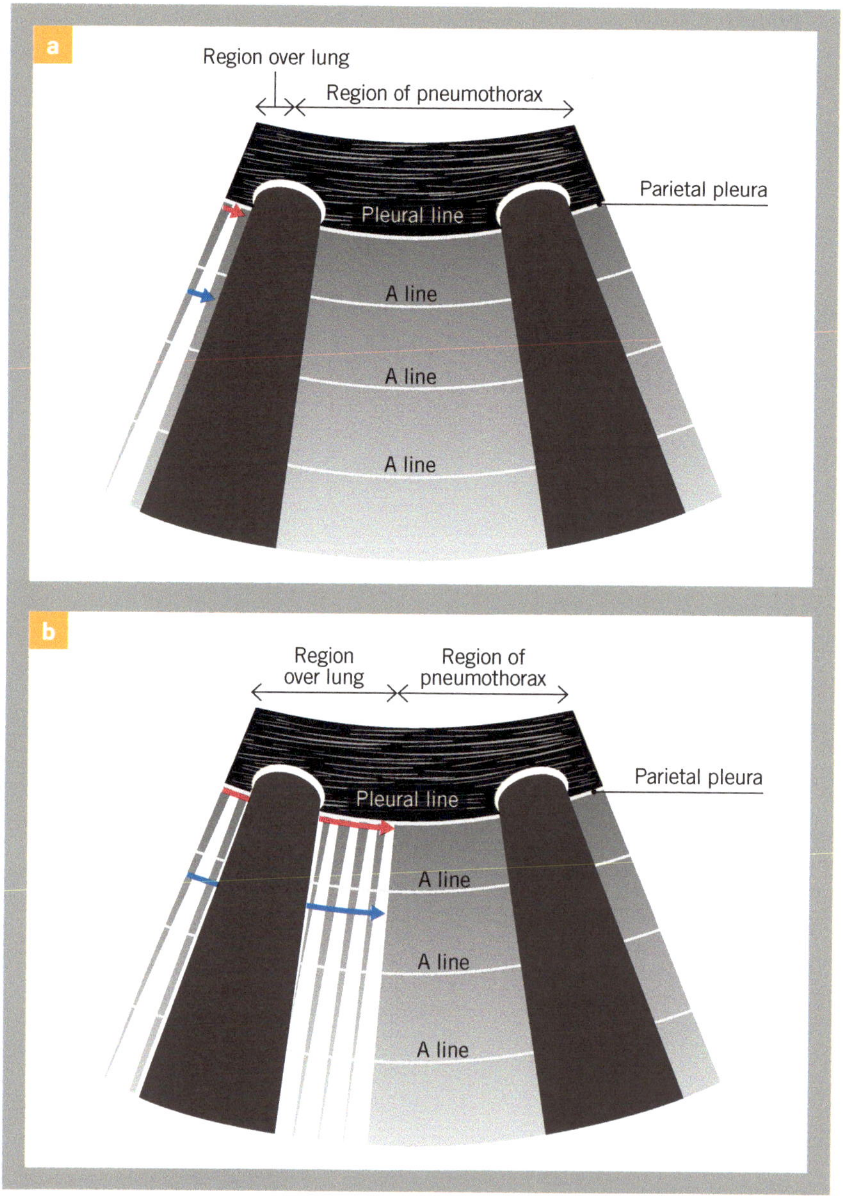

Figure 5. Ultrasound schematic images demonstrating a to-and-fro lung point in which the underlying lung tissue contains B lines. Start of inspiration. The leading edge of the lung is depicted by the B line on the left side of the image. Red arrowhead represents the lung surface in contact with the thoracic wall. Blue arrow represents the leading edge of a B line, which also represents the leading edge of the lung in this example (a). At the end of inspiration, the lung has reached its maximum expansion and begins to decrease in size during expiration. This will cause the lung to retreat to the size depicted in image a. Lung sliding advances and retreats with inspiration and expiration respectively, creates the to-and-fro partial lung slide. A divergent lung point is also possible to identify with B lines (not shown) (b).

It is possible to crudely estimate the degree of pneumothorax by dividing the thoracic wall into thirds and noting where the lung point occurs vertically along the thoracic wall (Fig. 6). Although tracking the movement of the lung point serially over time may be helpful at monitoring the progression or resolution of pneumothorax, the decision to perform thoracocentesis should be based on clinical findings and patient assessment, not on the location of the lung point. If the lung point is tracked it should be identified with the patient in the same position, ideally standing or sternal, each time. Rechecking PLUS for the presence of lung sliding and the lung point after thoracocentesis also provides a baseline from which to gauge further accumulation of air over time. If the pneumothorax is severe and the lung fails to recontact the thoracic wall, a lung point will not be found and lung sliding will be absent on that entire side of the thorax (Fig. 7). In this scenario, patients usually demonstrate signs of severe pneumothorax and therapeutic thoracocentesis should be performed immediately.

To find the lung point the operator moves the transducer from a region of pneumothorax towards the hilus of the lung. The starting point may be anywhere on the thorax where lung sliding is absent. Given the most sensitive sites for air to accumulate with pneumothorax are the caudodorsal regions in standing or sternal patients, and the widest point of the thoracic in the lateral patient, these are common starting points to begin a search for the lung point (see Chapter 2). The transducer is slid towards the lung hilus (usually cranially ventrally towards the elbow) from the area of pneumothorax, watching closely for the reappearance of lung sliding (Fig. 8).

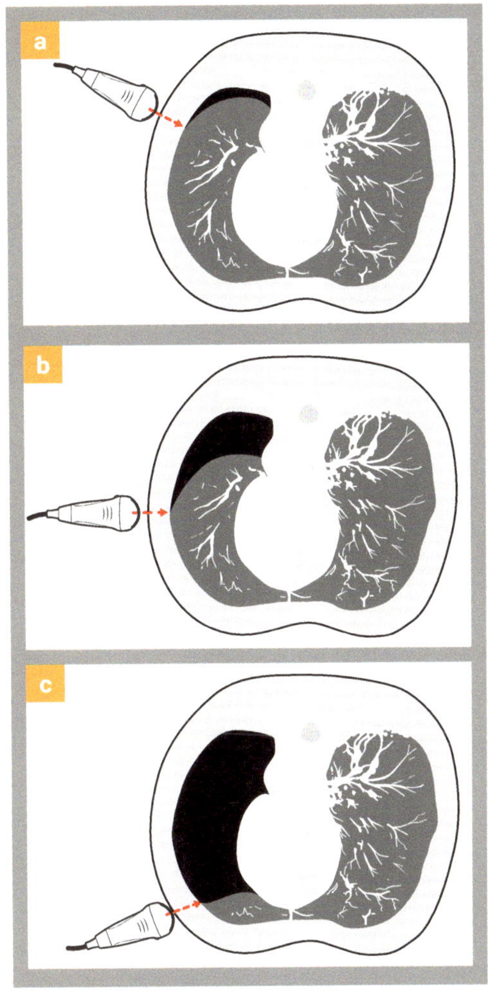

Figure 6. Computed tomography (CT) schematic images showing illustrated transducer locations. CT images are shown in short axis depicting transducer placement which can be used to track the size of pneumothorax. The red dotted arrow marks the lung point. The lung point is identified in the dorsal third of the thorax, indicating a smaller volume pneumothorax is present (a). The lung point is identified in the middle of the thorax, indicating a moderate volume pneumothorax is present (b). The lung point is identified in the ventral third of the thorax, indicating a large volume pneumothorax is present (c). The indication for thoracocentesis should be based on clinical signs, not the location of the lung point.

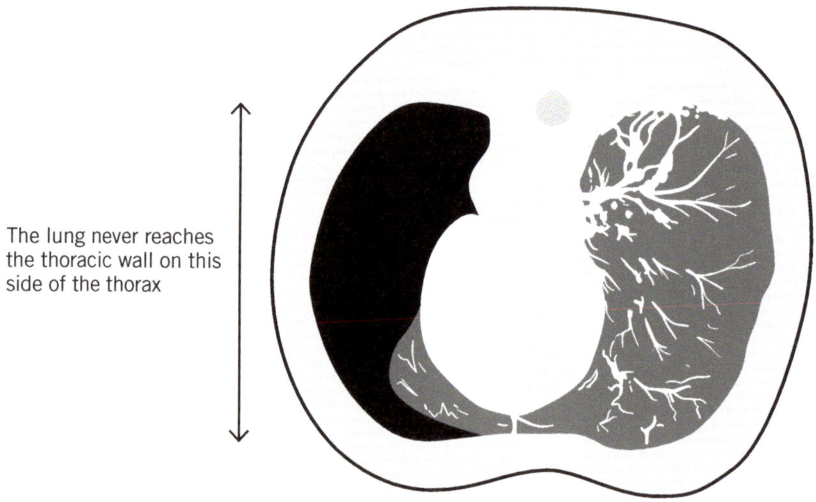

Figure 7. CT image of a massive pneumothorax where the lung fails to contact the lateral thoracic wall at any point on the left side of the CT image. In this case, both lung sliding and the lung point will not be detectable anywhere on the left side of the thoracic wall.

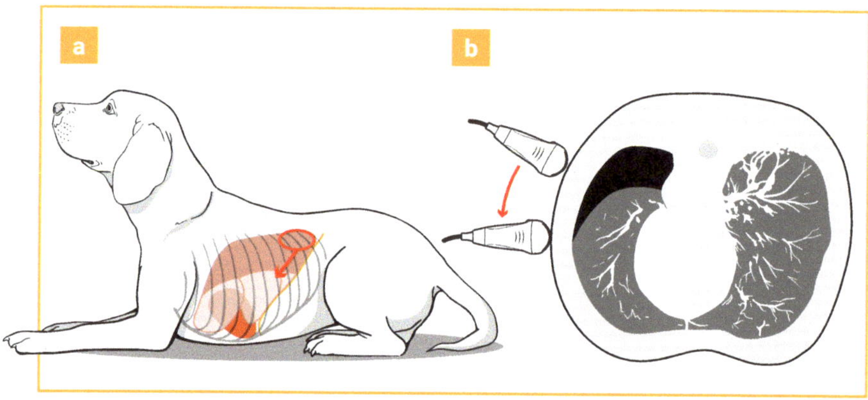

Figure 8. Schematic and computed tomography (CT) image indicating how the lung point can be identified. When the transducer is situated over an area of the thorax where no lung sliding is identified and pneumothorax is suspected the transducer should be slid from the area of absent lung sliding, in a cranial ventral region, towards the elbow (a). CT image showing movement of the transducer from an area where there is an absence of lung sliding to the lung point (b).

In some situations, the sonographer will move from an area where there is an absence of lung sliding (transducer is over pneumothorax) to an area where there is lung sliding (transducer is completely over aerated lung during the entire respiratory cycle [Fig. 9]). In this situation, the actual lung point may not have been identified, but moving from the absence of lung sliding to an obvious lung slide with supporting history and other clinical findings is sufficient to diagnose pneumothorax. This is particularly true given the lung sliding is usually more obvious in the caudodorsal lung regions (more lung sliding) than the cranioventral regions (less lung sliding). Therefore in a standing/sternal patient, finding an obvious lung slide cranioventrally with the absence of lung sliding caudodorsally is opposite to what is typically expected in healthy animals and should raise suspicion of pneumothorax (Chapter 3).

If the sonographic findings are uncertain, the opposite side of the thorax should be compared for the presence or absence of lung sliding, and the curtain sign should be evaluated for asynchronous or double curtain signs (see below), which is easier and faster for some sonographers to assess than lung sliding and the lung point.

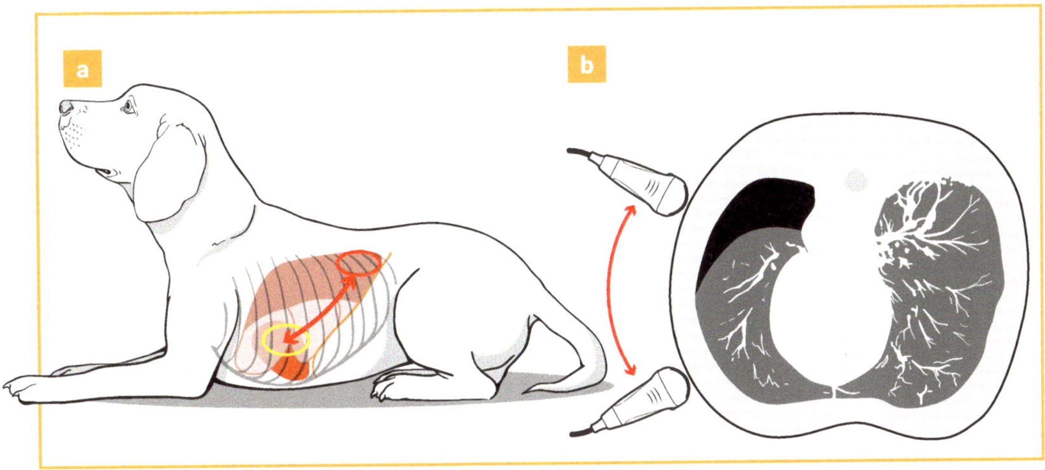

Figure 9. Schematic image indicating movement of the transducer back and forth from an area where there is no lung to an area where there is lung. Sliding the transducer back and forth form the absence to the presence of lung sliding indicates pneumothorax, even though the lung point itself was not identified (a). Computed tomography (CT) image showing movement of the transducer back and forth between pneumothorax and lung, which will result in the absence and appearance of lung sliding respectively (b).

Key concepts of lung point

- The lung point is an incomplete lung slide and is identified where the lung recontacts the thoracic wall; it is considered pathognomonic for pneumothorax.
- The lung point is visible when the transducer is positioned over a portion of sonographically visible aerated expanding lung (incomplete lung sliding visible) and simultaneously over free pleural air (lung sliding not visible).
- The lung point can appear differently depending on where and how it contacts the thoracic wall within the ultrasound image, and if the underlying lung is dry or contains sonographically visible lung pathology.
- Recognizing the return of lung sliding ventrally from a more dorsal position without lung sliding is indicative of pneumothorax.
- Concluding B lines always rule out pneumothorax can be misleading, as they may also be seen with the lung point.
- Lung sliding is used to both rule out and confirm pneumothorax; when it is present along the entire pleural line it rules out pneumothorax, when it is partial and only visible intermittently as seen with the lung point, it confirms the presence of pneumothorax.
- The sonographer has to carefully assess if lung sliding is complete or incomplete to avoid the error of concluding the presence of lung sliding rules out pneumothorax.

Abnormal pneumothorax-induced abdominal curtain signs: asynchronous and double curtain signs

Two abnormal pneumothorax-induced curtain signs have been documented in dogs with pneumothorax; asynchronous and double curtain signs. Although further research is required to determine the sensitivity and specificity of abnormal curtain signs to detect pneumothorax, it has been suggested that it may be more sensitive and specific than the lung point for diagnosis of small to medium volume pneumothorax in companion animals[5].

An advantage of assessing the curtain sign in the patient with rapid shallow breathing, often the case in patients with pneumothorax, is the ultrasound image can be frozen. Thus, the stored video loop can be viewed by scrolling back several frames, which allows the curtain sign to be visualized at a slower speed. This often makes it easier to determine if normal and/or abnormal abdominal curtain signs are present. Freezing and scrolling back through frames at a slower rate is less helpful for assessment of lung sliding or the lung point as it is the dynamic nature of the lungs sliding across the thoracic wall which creates the sonographic shimmering of lung sliding; the shimmer is less visible when an ultrasound image is frozen and video loops assessed at a slower speed. When a double curtain sign is present it is also possible to diagnose pneumothorax with a still image in some situations.

In healthy individuals, the abdominal curtain sign moves caudally on inspiration with other visible abdominal contents at a similar rate; the movement of the vertical edge and abdominal contents is therefore synchronous (Fig. 10; see video 3.7 in Chapter 3). Although the abdominal curtain sign may not be visible as it slides under ribs or it slides caudally out of the ultrasound image, it is always present in healthy animals.

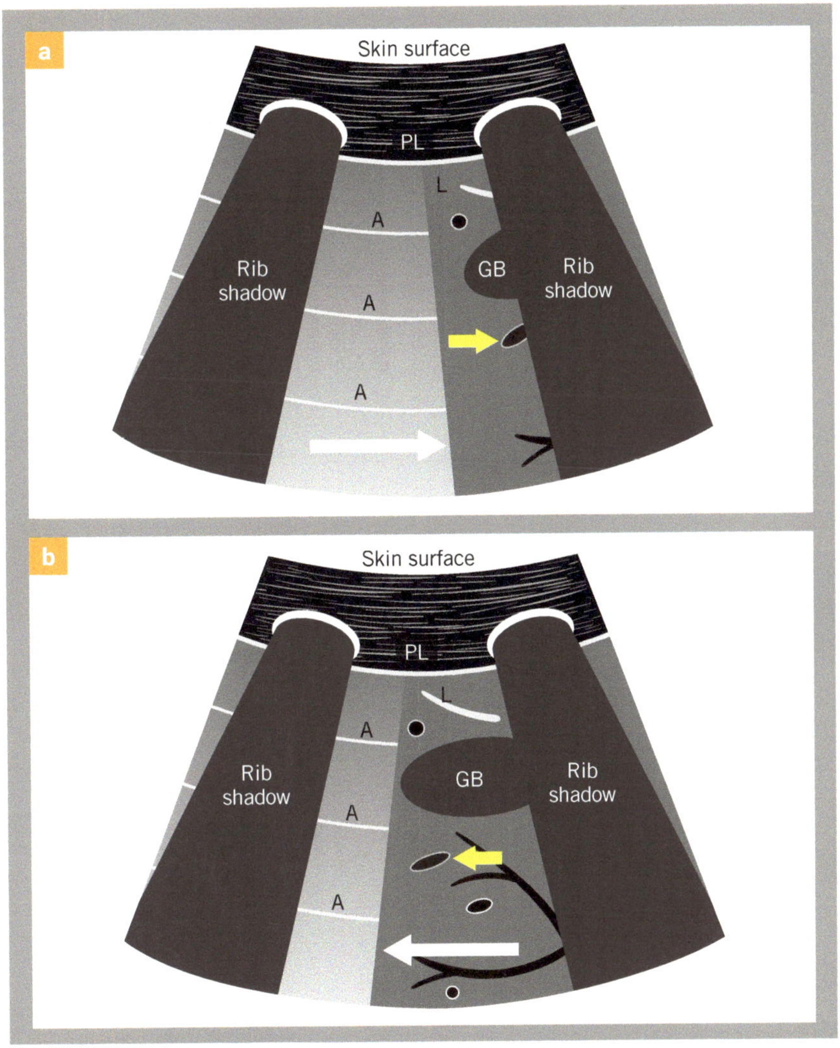

Figure 10. Schematic ultrasound images of the normal abdominal curtain sign with the transducer transverse to the ribs and the marker directed cranial. During inspiration the curtain sign and abdominal contents (yellow arrow) are shown sliding caudally in sync with each other (a). During expiration the curtain sign and abdominal contents are shown moving cranially together (b). The liver and gallbladder, hepatic and portal veins are shown. A; A lines, PL; pleural line, L; liver, GB; gallbladder.

In the absence of pneumothorax, the location of the cranial aspect of the costophrenic recess changes with respirations, moving caudally on inspiration as the diaphragm contracts and the lung slides caudally to replace it (Fig. 11; right side of CT images). The caudal border of the costophrenic recess is fixed and represents the reflection of the parietal pleura from the thoracic wall onto the diaphragm. In the absence of pneumothorax, the lung will slide into the costophrenic recess as the diaphragm contracts, resulting in the curtain sign moving caudally on inspiration. As the lung slides into the costophrenic recess it separates the diaphragm and abdomen from the thoracic wall, preventing abdominal structures from being sonographically visible. In the presence of pneumothorax, free air in the pleural space is present cranial to the costophrenic recess and small pockets of pleural air can be seen within the costophrenic recess (Fig. 11; left side of CT images).

With pneumothorax-induced double curtain signs, two soft tissue-to-air interfaces (a cranial and caudal interface) are visible within the same sonographic window (Fig. 12). A double

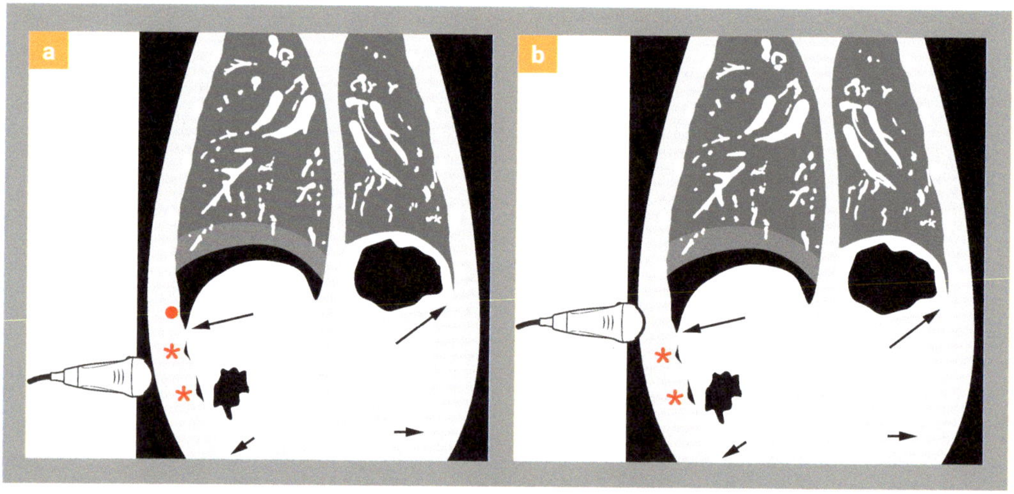

Figure 11. Schematic computed tomography (CT) image demonstrating a pneumothorax on the left side of a dog. The long black arrow represents the cranial aspect of the costophrenic recess and the short black arrow represent the caudal aspect of the costophrenic recess where the diaphragm attaches to the thoracic wall. If the transducer is placed between the two asterisks, two pneumothorax induced curtain signs (air soft tissue interfaces) will be seen; the double curtain sign. If the transducer is placed between the cranial asterisk and the red dot, a pneumothorax induced curtain sign is visible at the location of the long black arrow. When the patient inspires the diaphragm contracts, causing any visible abdominal contents to move caudally, while at the same time the thoracic wall moves outward. Because there is no lung to prevent the abdominal contents from coming into contact with the thoracic wall cranial to long black arrow, the negative pleural pressure created during inspiration allows the diaphragm and abdominal contents to move laterally into contact with the thoracic wall, giving the impression the curtain sign is moving cranially. This creates the asynchronous curtain sign. If the ultrasound beam is moved more cranially (level of the red circle), it will be situated over a region of only pneumothorax. During inspiration the abdominal contents may "suddenly appear" as the diaphragm is pulled laterally into contact with the thoracic wall where previously only pneumothorax and the bat sign with absent lung sliding were visible. This creates an appearing and disappearing double curtain sign.

curtain sign can be seen when the transducer is placed over a region of the costophrenic recess that contains trapped air at two different locations (Figs. 11a and 12), or it can suddenly appear during inspiration if the diaphragm and abdominal contents are pulled laterally into contact with the thoracic wall where previously only pneumothorax and the bat sign with absent lung sliding were visible (Figs. 11b and 12). Similar to the divergent lung point, the double curtain sign may suddenly appear at a central point within the ultrasound image and expand bidirectionally (Fig. 12; video 4.8). Although the normal abdominal curtain sign may not be visible when it slides under ribs (obscured by rib shadows) or extends beyond the caudal border of the ultrasound image, it is always visible as a vertical air edge artifact. In contrast, the abnormal double curtain sign can suddenly appear and disappear within the ultrasound image without passing under ribs or sliding caudally out of the ultrasound image (Fig. 12).

With a pneumothorax-induced asynchronous curtain sign the vertical air edge artifact moves cranially, or fails to move at all, while the abdominal contents move caudally (Fig. 13; video 4.9). The curtain and the abdominal content are asynchronous to each other. This is believed to occur when pleural air is present lateral and cranial to the diaphragm and there is no lung present to slide into the costophrenic recess when the patient inspires, allowing the soft tissue structures to move laterally into contact with the thoracic wall (Fig. 11b).

Hint: assess both the direction of the curtain sign and abdominal contents with regards to each other to decide if they move in the same or opposite directions during the respiratory cycle.

QR
Video 4.9.
Asynchronous curtains.

QR
Video 4.8.
Double curtain signs.

QR
Video 4.10.
Mixed abnormal curtains.

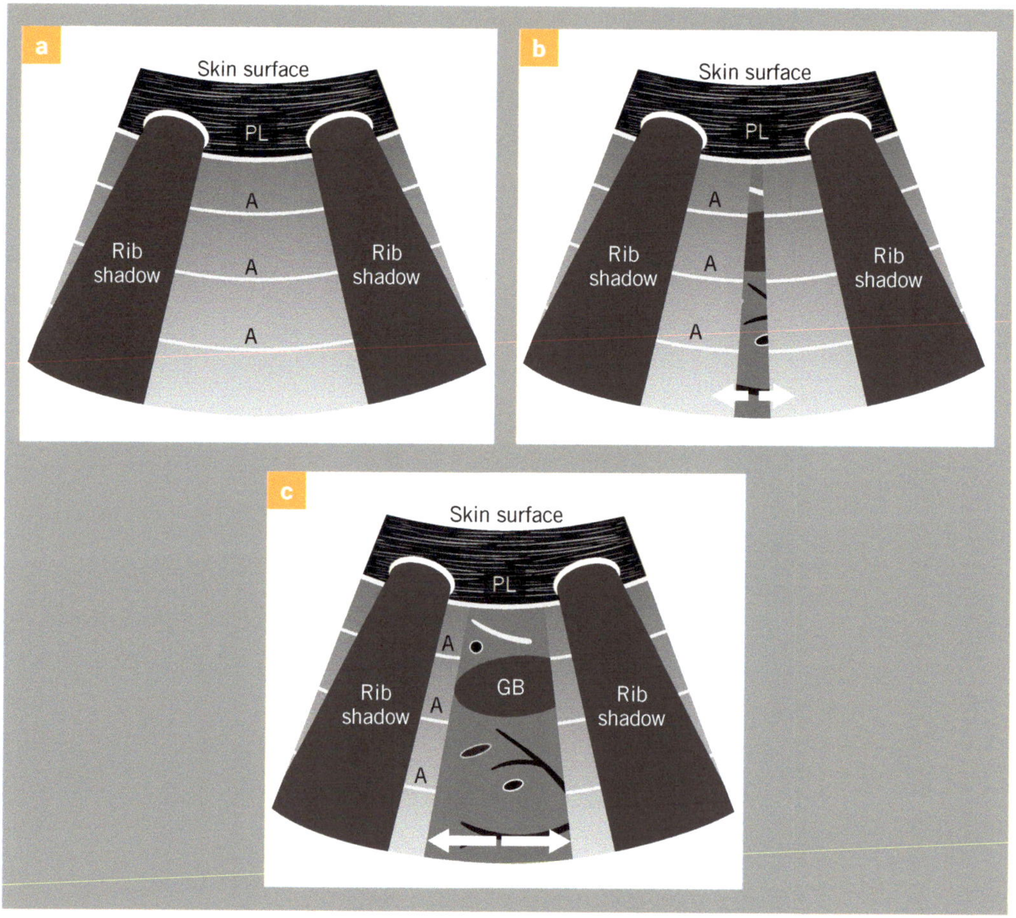

Figure 12. Schematic ultrasound images of a pneumothorax-induced double curtain sign with the transducer transverse to the ribs and the marker directed cranial. (a) In this example, the transducer is situated just cranial to the costophrenic recess in the caudal region of the thorax. Only A lines are present and there is no lung sliding visible. There is no curtain sign in this image as the transducer is over air in the pleural space (pneumothorax) giving rise to the classic bat sign (a). During inspiration the curtain sign is abnormal as it suddenly appears in the centre of the ultrasound image and expands both cranially and caudally (white arrows); soft tissue abdominal contents suddenly "break" into the reverberation artifact of A lines and expand bidirectionally (b). The visible soft tissue structures and both edges of the curtain sign may grow until end expiration is reached, at which point the process reverses (c). It is also possible to see the double curtain sign through respiration which would be represented by Figure 12b–c. Other variation of the abnormal curtain sign can also exist which are not shown here. The liver and gallbladder, hepatic and portal veins are shown. A; A lines, PL; pleural line, L; liver, GB; gallbladder.

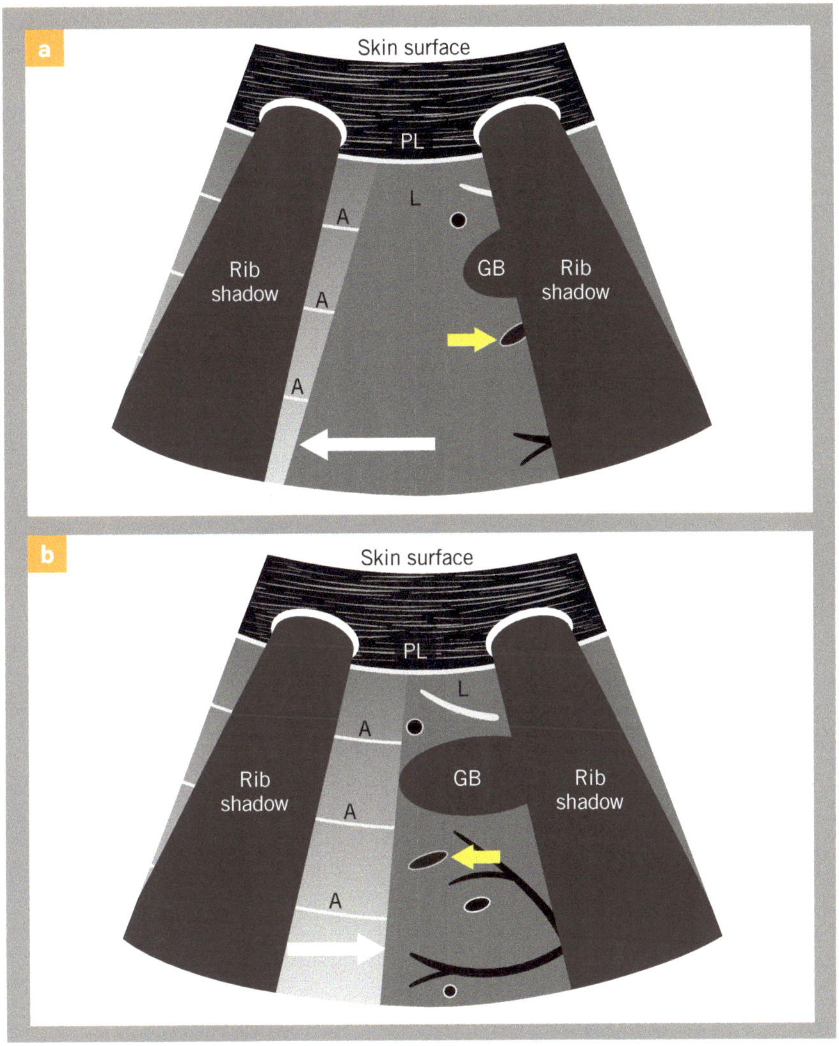

Figure 13. Schematic ultrasound images of a pneumothorax-induced asynchronous abdominal curtain sign with the transducer transverse to the ribs and the marker directed cranial. During inspiration the curtain sign is abnormal as it moves cranially while the abdominal contents (yellow arrow) still slide caudally during inspiration; the two are asynchronous (a). During expiration the curtain sign moves caudal while the abdominal contents move cranial. The liver and gallbladder, hepatic and portal veins are shown (b). A; A lines, P; pleural line, L; liver, GB; gallbladder.

In standing patients with pneumothorax, the curtain sign is often normal in the ventral regions of the thorax, with asynchronous and double curtain signs being identified more dorsally on the thorax. Therefore, it is possible to see variations of the curtain sign on the same side of the thorax of patients with pneumothorax as one sweeps the transducer dorsally and ventrally along the curtain sign with the transducer in perpendicular orientation to the ribs (video 4.10). This is helpful to sonographers as sweeping from an area where a subtle asynchronous curtain sign is present to an obvious double curtain sign or ventrally to a region where the curtain sign is normal helps confirm the diagnosis of pneumothorax.

Key concepts of abnormal abdominal curtain signs

- Asynchronous and double curtain signs have been identified in dogs with pneumothorax.
- In the dyspneic patient with asynchronous or double curtain signs and concurrent supporting history and clinical findings of pneumothorax, thoracocentesis is indicated.
- It is possible to find normal and abnormal curtain signs on the same side of the thorax in patients with pneumothorax if the transducer is swept from ventral to dorsal.
- The transducer should be swept ventrally and dorsally along the curtain sign to assess and compare it at different locations.
- In patients with rapid shallow breathing, the ultrasound image can be frozen and the stored video loop viewed by scrolling backwards and forwards allowing the curtain sign to be visualized at a slower speed.

Table 1. The five key criteria to evaluate when assessing pneumothorax at the transducer site.

Criteria that rule out pneumothorax	Criteria that rule in pneumothorax
▪ Complete lung sliding ▪ B lines/lung consolidation ▪ Lung pulse	▪ Abnormal abdominal curtain signs (asynchronous/double) ▪ Lung point

THE ROLE OF M MODE TO DIAGNOSE PNEUMOTHORAX

Given lung sliding is sometimes difficult to identify with B mode, motion mode or M mode ultrasound has been used to document the presence or absence of pneumothorax in human patients[6]. Although it is occasionally used in veterinary patients, studies documenting the value of M mode for assessment of pneumothorax in companion animals are lacking. Keeping distressed dogs and cats calm and still, which is required with M mode, can be very challenging; this may explain why M mode is not utilized as often as B mode for detection of pneumothorax in companion animals.

With M mode the pleural line is visible as a bright horizontal white line while the soft tissues of the thoracic wall above the pleural line appear as horizontal linear lines of variable echogenicity; they appear linear as they have relatively little movement throughout the respiratory cycle of patients with or without pneumothorax (Fig. 14). In contrast, the lung, which appears below the pleural line, varies in appearance between healthy patients and patients with pneumothorax. When an animal with healthy lungs breathes, motion within the lung changes the lung artifacts that return to the machine, creating a speckled appearance like grains of sand beneath the pleural line (Fig. 14; video 4.11). This creates the image of a "seashore" where soft tissues above the pleural line appear linear like waves, while the lung below the pleural line appears as sand at a beach (seashore sign). When a pneumothorax is present, there will be minimal to no motion detected above or below the pleural line by M mode as the lung is separated from the thoracic wall and not visible through air. This creates an M mode image referred to as the "barcode or stratosphere sign" where the soft tissue structures above the pleural line appear similar to the region of pneumothorax below the pleural line (Fig. 14; video 4.12).

QR

Video 4.11.
M mode seashore sign.

QR

Video 4.12.
M mode pneumotorax.

Healthy lung has been described as having a "sand on the beach" or "seashore sign" appearance with M mode. In the presence of pneumothorax, a "barcode or stratosphere sign" is created.

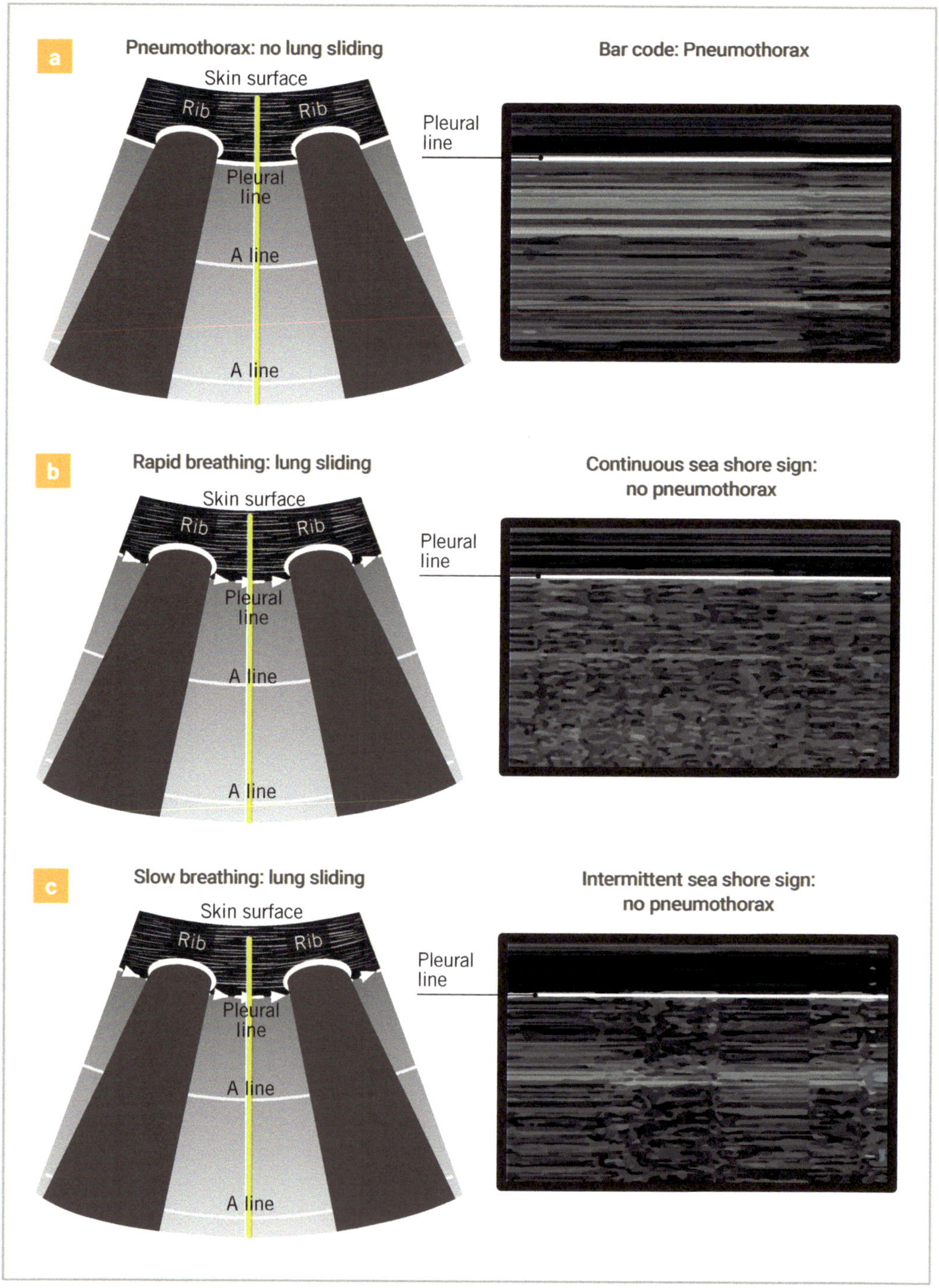

Figure 14. Schematic and M mode ultrasound images of a patient that has pneumothorax (a) with a barcode sign, no pneumothorax but rapid shallow breathing and a continuous seashore sign (b) and slow breathing intermittent seashore sign (c).

If there is movement of the patient or the transducer then speckling similar to the "sand on a beach" sign may occur; however, this is due to motion artifact. It can be differentiated from healthy lung because the speckling originates above the pleural line with motion artifact and below the pleural line with healthy lungs. Motion artifact may obscure the barcode sign from being visible in cases of pneumothorax; therefore, the patient and the transducer must be kept still to use M mode accurately.

Common mistakes to avoid when diagnosing pneumothorax

There are several common mistakes to avoid when searching for pneumothorax:

- Concluding that any evidence of lung sliding rules out pneumothorax:
  - Incomplete or intermittent lung sliding is visible with all lung points, which confirm the diagnosis of pneumothorax.
- Concluding that the absence of lung sliding confirms pneumothorax:
  - Lung sliding can be difficult to find in some healthy patients and becomes more challenging in patients with respiratory disease.
- Concluding that the presence of B lines always rules out pneumothorax:
  - B lines can be seen with a lung point if the underlying lung has sonographically visible pathology.
- Concluding that the presence of A lines rules out pneumothorax:
  - A lines are present with healthy lung and pneumothorax.
- Mistaking Z lines for B lines:
  - Z lines have no significance and can be present in both healthy lung and pneumothorax.
- Failing to assess the most gravity-independent (highest) sites:
  - Air rises and these sites are the most sensitive regions to locate or rule out pneumothorax.
- Failing to evaluate the abdominal curtain sign:
  - Abnormal abdominal curtain signs confirm pneumothorax and may be easier to find and interpret than searching for a lung point.

DIAGNOSTIC APPROACH

Transducer orientation/selection

A microconvex curvilinear transducer is used by the authors. A linear array transducer and phased array transducer can be used to assess lung sliding, although there are no studies in veterinary medicine to suggest an advantage of these transducers over the microconvex for diagnosis of pneumothorax.

In general, the depth is set at 2–6 cm, depending on the patient's body condition score; obese patients require a deeper setting, thin patients a shallower setting. A good rule of thumb is to place the pleural line at approximately the 1/3 to 1/2 line of the ultrasound image. Shallower depths may make lung sliding easier to visualize.

Transducer settings are adjusted to make the pleural line appear grainy; the grainier the pleural line, the easier it is to identify lung sliding. See normal lung sliding (Chapter 3) for general tricks regarding transducer manipulation to make the pleural line grainier and lung sliding easier to visualize.

- With pneumothorax air accumulates at the most gravity-independent (highest) sites/pleural borders, which change with patient positioning.
- In a standing or sternally recumbent patient the caudodorsal border is the most sensitive location to find smaller volume pneumothorax.
- In a laterally recumbent patient, the widest point of the thorax is the most sensitive site to find smaller volume pneumothorax.
- It is important to not compromise patient safety: if the history and signalment are supportive of pneumothorax, along with other clinical findings (e.g. absence of breath sounds in a trauma patient), immediate therapeutic thoracocentesis is indicated.

Sonographic technique to identify pneumothorax

Patient position affects where the air will rise and, therefore, the most sensitive site to locate pneumothorax (Fig. 15).

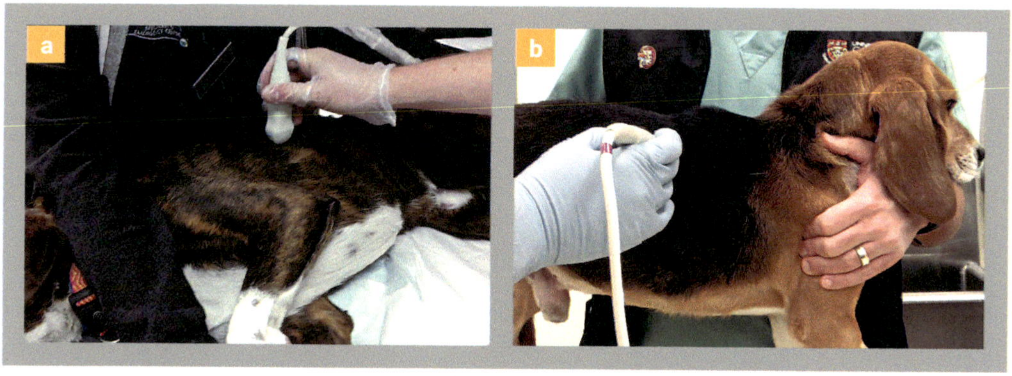

Figure 15. Images showing where to place the transducer to find the most sensitive sonographic sites for diagnosis of pneumothorax based on patient position. Image of a dog in lateral recumbency with the transducer situated over the widest point of the thorax (a). Image of a dog with the transducer at the most caudodorsal location (b).

Standing or sternal patient

The most caudodorsal regions should be assessed to identify smaller volume pneumothorax:

1. Start by placing the transducer behind the thoracic limb, roughly at the widest point of the thorax or 2/3 of the way up the thorax (see Fig. 6 in Chapter 2). With experience and knowledge of the sonographically-defined pleura and lung borders (see Chapter 1), the operator can start closer to the caudodorsal border.
2. Assess the pleural line at this starting location for the presence or absence of lung sliding (Fig. 16; videos 4.1 and 4.2); moderate to large volume pneumothorax will result in the absence of lung sliding at the starting location.

- If lung sliding is absent, pneumothorax should be suspected and a search undertaken for the lung point, return of lung sliding, and/or abnormal curtain signs.
- If complete lung sliding is present, pneumothorax is ruled out at the starting transducer location (moderate to large volume pneumothorax is unlikely on that side of the thorax). However, pneumothorax has not been ruled out at the more sensitive caudodorsal location:
  - Slide the transducer caudally until the curtain sign is identified (caudal PLUS border), and then follow the curtain sign dorsally until the pleural line disappears in the hypaxial/sublumbar muscles (dorsal PLUS border).

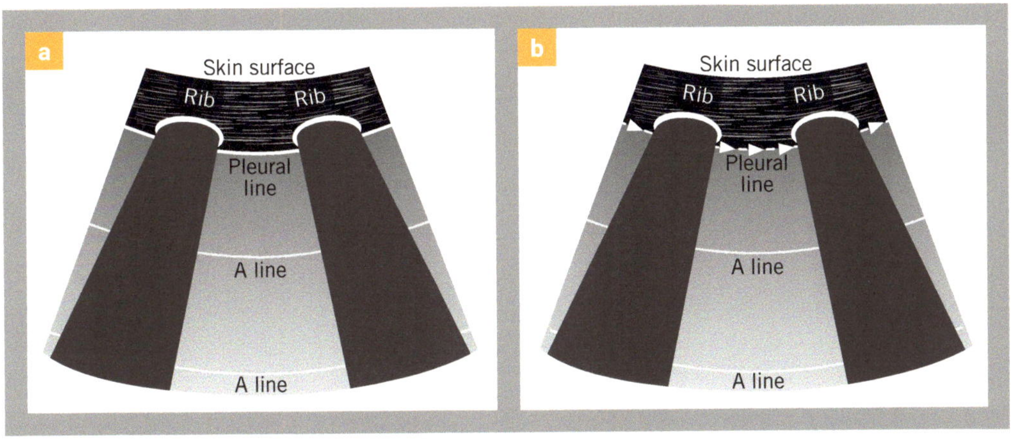

Figure 16. Schematic ultrasound images demonstrating the absence of lung sliding due to pneumothorax (a) and the presence of lung sliding (b) in a healthy animal. Both images are very similar demonstrating the same soft tissue structures, ribs, rib shadows (black) and A lines. A soft tissue-to-air interface is present at the pleural line in healthy lungs and in patients with pneumothorax. Lung sliding, lung pulse and B lines are absent in figure 16a where the pleura line is only composed of the parietal pleura, and lung sliding is present in figure 16b, depicted by the dotted line and arrow heads which represent the visceral pleura is in contact with and sliding along the parietal pleura. The presence of a lung pulse and/or B lines in figure 16b (not shown) would also rule out pneumothorax.

- Assess the curtain sign as normal or abnormal during the entire process of moving to the most caudodorsal site (see Fig. 9, Chapter 2; see videos 3.7, 4.8, 4.9 and 4.10).
  - If the curtain sign is assessed as an asynchronous curtain sign or double curtain sign (see below) pneumothorax should be suspected and thoracocentesis performed depending on the clinical signs and supporting evidence for pneumothorax.
  - If the curtain sign is normal over the length it is scanned, pneumothorax is unlikely. However, lung sliding can be assessed at the most caudodorsal site if the sonographer has a strong suspicion for smaller volume pneumothorax.
- If lung sliding is absent at the most caudodorsal site, pneumothorax should be suspected but cannot be sonographically confirmed based on the absence of lung sliding alone.
  - An abnormal curtain sign and/or the lung point should be identified to definitively confirm the diagnosis of pneumothorax.
  - If the history and signalment are supportive of pneumothorax, along with other clinical findings (e.g. absence of breath sounds), thoracocentesis and patient stabilization takes precedence over searching for the lung point or abnormal curtain signs.
- If complete lung sliding is present at the most caudodorsal site (most non-gravity dependent highest point), pneumothorax is ruled out on that side of the thorax and the other side of the thorax should be evaluated.

Laterally positioned patient

1. The search for a pneumothorax is very similar to that described for the sternal patient, however the widest non-gravity dependent region of the thorax is the most sensitive site for pneumothorax to occur in the laterally recumbent patient, and is the preferred site to assess for the presence or absence of lung sliding. Assessment of the curtain sign is the same regardless of patient positioning.
2. If complete lung sliding is present at the widest non gravity dependent point of the thorax of a patient in lateral recumbency, pneumothorax is ruled out on that side of the thorax and the other side of the thorax should be evaluated.
3. If lung sliding is absent at the widest non gravity dependent point of the thorax, pneumothorax should be suspected and a lung point (see below) or presence of an abnormal curtain sign should be assessed.

Regardless of patient position, be sure to check both sides of the thorax for pneumothorax. Comparing the two sides of the thorax for the presence or absence of lung sliding, lung point and curtain signs can be beneficial and build confidence in the diagnosis if pneumothorax is unilateral.

PITFALLS

In the authors' experience, failure to assess the most gravity independent pleural border, mistaking the lung point for lung sliding, mistaking Z lines for B lines, mistaking curtain sign movement for lung sliding, and not assessing the curtain sign are the most common reasons why sonographers fail to detect pneumothorax using ultrasound.

Massive pneumothorax is sonographically challenging to diagnose as the lung point will not be visible if the lungs fail to recontact the thoracic wall. In addition, abnormal abdominal curtain signs have not yet been evaluated in cases with massive pneumothorax. Therefore, it is not worth spending time looking for these findings in the markedly dyspneic patient suspected to have massive pneumothorax.

There is limited research on sonographically identifying pneumothorax in cats; the sensitivity and specificity using the criteria to rule in our rule out pneumothorax in cats has not yet been established.

SUMMARY

Scanning the thorax in a systemic fashion by finding the pleural space and lung border and asking binary questions enhances the chances of finding pneumothorax. There are both rule out and rule in findings that need to be evaluated in assessing a patient for pneumothorax. Increasing sensitivity and specificity for assessing pneumothorax can be achieved by:

- Scanning the most gravity independent sites, which change with patient position.
- Looking for abnormal curtain signs.
- Searching for the lung point/return of lung sliding.

REFERENCES

1. Lisciandro GR, Lagutchik MS, Mann KA, et al. Evaluation of a thoracic focused assessment with sonography for trauma (TFAST) protocol to detect pneumothorax and concurrent thoracic injury in 145 traumatized dogs. *J Vet Emerg Crit Care*, 2008, 18:258.
2. Armenise A, Boysen RS, Rudloff E, Neri L, et al. Veterinary-focused assessment with sonography for trauma-airway, breathing, circulation, disability and exposure: a prospective observational study in 64 canine trauma patients. *J Small Anim Pract*, 2019, 60(3):173–182.
3. Cole L, Pivetta M, Humm K. Diagnostic accuracy of a lung ultrasound protocol (Vet BLUE) for detection of pleural fluid, pneumothorax and lung pathology in dogs and cats. *J Small Anim Pract*, 2021, 62(3):178–186.
4. Walters AM, O'Brien MA, Selmic LE, et al. Evaluation of the agreement between focused assessment with sonography for trauma (AFAST/TFAST) and computed tomography in dogs and cats with recent trauma. *J Vet Emerg Crit Care (San Antonio)*. 2018, 28(5):429–435.
5. Boysen S, McMurray J, Gommeren K. Abnormal Curtain Signs Identified With a Novel Lung Ultrasound Protocol in Six Dogs With Pneumothorax. *Front Vet Sci*, 2019, 6:291
6. Lichtenstein D. Lung ultrasound in the critically ill. *Curr Opin Crit Care*, 2014, 20(3):315–322.

05

CLINICAL APPLICATIONS OF PLUS: IS THERE PLEURAL EFFUSION, YES/NO?

INTRODUCTION

Pleural effusion appears as hypoechoic accumulations separating the parietal and visceral pleura, and its appearance can vary depending on the cellularity of the effusion, transducer location, patient positioning, the quantity of fluid, and the presence of adhesions.

The sonographic accuracy to detect pleural effusion is relatively good and effusion is easier to diagnose than pneumothorax, but small amounts of pleural effusion can be missed[1-3]. Finding pleural effusion with PLUS leads to further diagnostic and therapeutic considerations. For instance, ultrasound-guided thoracocentesis would lead to improved patient stability if the fluid is sufficient to cause respiratory compromise, and analysis of the fluid may lead to an etiologic diagnosis.

Pleural effusion separates the visceral pleura from the parietal pleura resulting in a loss of lung sliding, however the visceral pleura is still visible as a hyperechoic white line (depth may have to be increased) because fluid transmits ultrasound beams (vs. pneumothorax where air is an enemy of ultrasound and, therefore, the visceral pleura cannot be seen when the transducer is placed directly over a region of pneumothorax) (Fig. 1; video 5.1).

Due to the effects of gravity, pleural effusion will accumulate in gravity-dependent (lowest) regions of the pleural space, often forming sharp angles, and tracking along and outlining the diaphragm (Fig. 2; video 5.2).

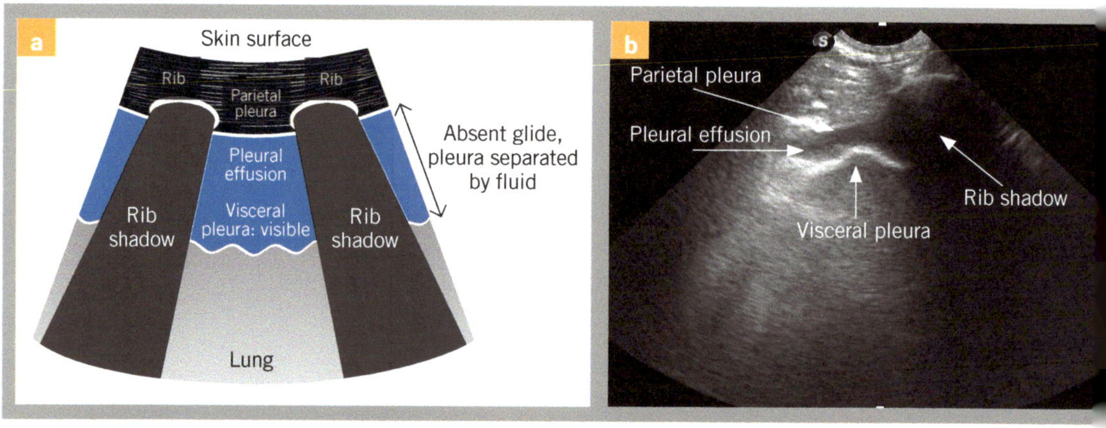

Figure 1. Schematic ultrasound image showing separation of the visceral pleura from the parietal pleura due to the presence of fluid in the pleural space (pleural effusion) with the transducer in perpendicular rib orientation. In this instance, the pleural line (solid white line) is composed of only the parietal pleura and, therefore, lung sliding is absent (i.e. the two pleura are not in contact). The lower curvilinear horizontal line represents the visceral pleura, which is separated from the parietal pleura by fluid. Fluid transmits ultrasound; therefore, the visceral pleura is visible (a). Ultrasound image of pleural effusion with the transducer in perpendicular orientation to the ribs. Both parietal and visceral pleura are visible because fluid is separating them. Fluid allows ultrasound beams to penetrate which allows the visualization of the visceral pleura. Although the visceral pleura is visible and will move with respirations, no lung sliding is present because the two pleura are separated (b).

QR
Video 5.1.
Perpendicular pleural effusion.

QR
Video 5.2.
PCS pleural with effusion consolidation.

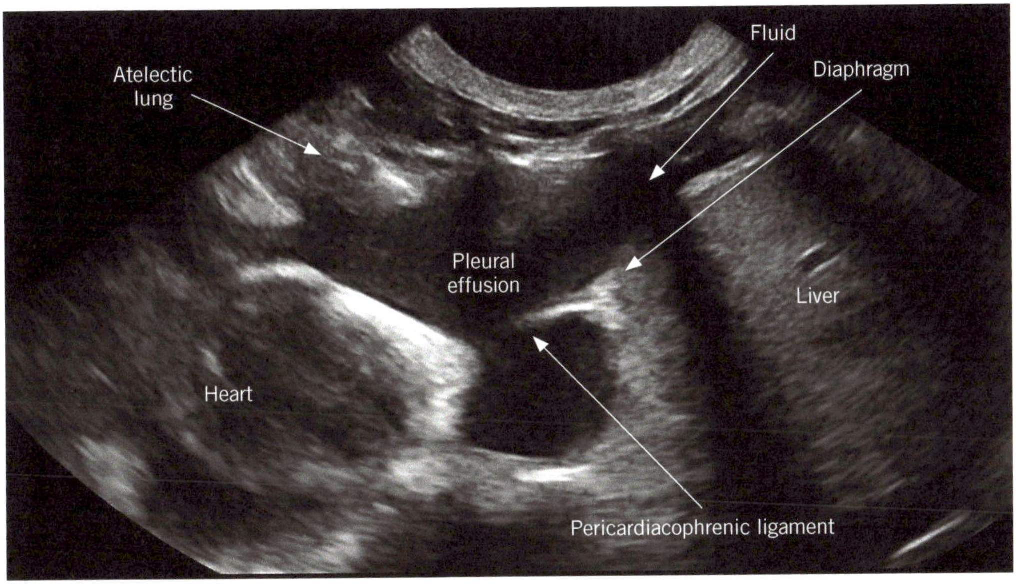

Figure 2. Pleural effusion in a sternal patient at the pericardiodiaphragmatic (PD) site, transducer in perpendicular rib orientation. Pleural effusion is affected by gravity and accumulates in the most gravity-dependent (lowest) sites of the pleural space. In this example, pleural effusion in a cat with feline infectious peritonitis (FIP) is seen at the PD site and the effusion forms angles with other structures. In addition, the pleural effusion is sufficient to track along (up and down) the diaphragm and fill the costophrenic recess. This ultrasound window is the key factor in determining if effusion is pericardial or pleural in nature, as pericardial effusion would be contained in the pericardial sac, curving away from the diaphragm and surrounding the heart.

QR
Video 5.3.
Pericardial effusion.

QR
Video 5.4.
Pericardiodiaphragmatic (PD) pleural effusion.

This is in contrast to pericardial effusion where the fluid will be contained within the pericardial sac and will follow the circular contour of the heart (Fig. 3; video 5.3).

Large quantities of pleural effusion are easily identified in patients in sternal recumbency in the ventral third of the thorax outlining the diaphragm and lungs and separating the parietal and visceral pleura at the pericardiodiaphragmatic (PD) window (Fig. 2; video 5.4). For patients in lateral recumbency, large pleural effusions can be easily visualized at the widest gravity-dependent portion (lowest) of the thorax.

Small quantities of pleural effusion can be missed in the sternal or standing patient, particularly when the transducer is only placed over the heart or situated at the costochondral junctions in perpendicular orientation to the ribs, as recommended in thoracic FAST protocols[3-4]. To identify smaller effusions, the transducer should be rotated into parallel orientation (marker dorsally) at the PD window or level the costochondral junction in a sternal/standing patient. As pleural fluid accumulates the lungs may become atelectatic, appearing as tissue-like structures "floating" within pleural effusions (Fig. 4; video 5.5).

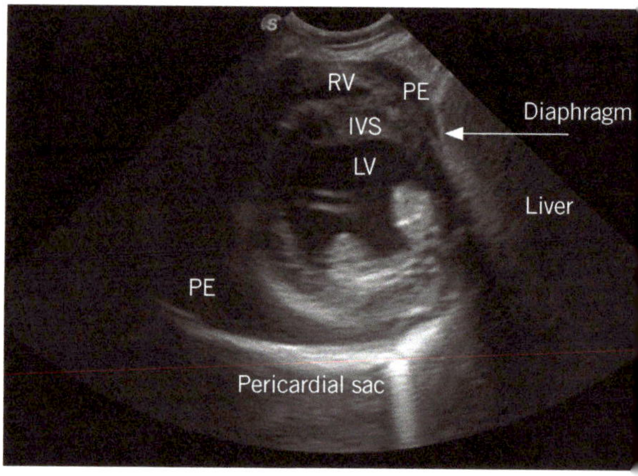

Figure 3. Pericardial effusion in a dog with transducer in perpendicular rib orientation at the pericardiodiaphragmatic (PD) window. The fluid is contained inside the pericardium and can be seen curving around the heart along the contours of the pericardial sac as well as curving away from the diaphragm. IVS: interventricular septum; LV: left ventricle; RV: right ventricle; PE: pericardial effusion.

Atelectatic lung in pleural effusion is termed the "jellyfish" sign in human medicine (Lichtenstein, 2005).

Healthy lung is not seen in normal patients (air is an enemy of ultrasound) but when pleural effusion causes the lung to collapse, the lung will have a soft tissue appearance due to the lack of aerated lung (see Chapter 7); hence, it is visible as tissue within pleural effusion because ultrasound beams can traverse the fluid and atelectic lung (video 5.2).

Pleural effusion can only be ruled in or out at the location the transducer is placed on the thorax. It is therefore essential to assess the most sensitive sites for pleural effusion to avoid missing smaller quantities of fluid.

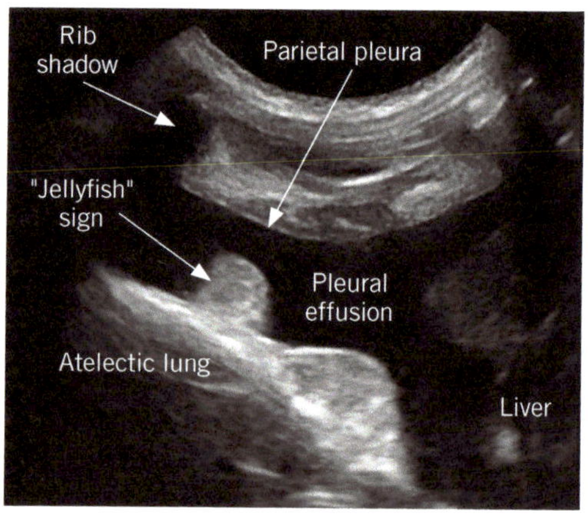

Figure 4. Image of an atelectatic lung ("jellyfish" sign) just dorsal to the pericardiodiaphragmatic (PD) window at the thoracoabdominal interface, transducer in perpendicular orientation to the ribs. When air is removed from lung, it adopts a tissue-like-pattern on ultrasound, meaning it becomes visible because ultrasound beams can now be transmitted through it (see Chapter 7, lung consolidation). Sometimes the atelectatic lung will move back and forth and have the appearance of a "jellyfish".

QR
Video 5.5.
"Jellyfish" sign.

Key concepts

- Pleural effusion accumulates in gravity-dependent (lowest) regions of the pleural space.
- When pleural effusion separates the two pleura, lung sliding is not present.
- The appearance of pleural effusion varies depending on transducer orientation, quantity of fluid, location of the fluid, cellularity and adhesions, and patient positioning.
- Atelectatic lung can create a "jellyfish" sign.
- Assessing the PD window allows differentiation of pleural from pericardial effusion.
- Large amounts of pleural effusion are easily identified in the gravity-dependent (lowest) regions of the thorax regardless of transducer orientation or patient position. Nevertheless, patient position must be accounted for to locate the gravity-dependent regions.
- Small amounts of pleural effusion are often missed ventrally and can be identified with the transducer in parallel orientation to the ribs.

CRITERIA TO DIAGNOSE PLEURAL EFFUSION

The presence of fluid between the parietal and visceral pleura eliminates lung sliding and confirms pleural effusion.

Although the visceral pleura (lung surface) may be visible deep to the effusion and may still move with respiration, one of the key criteria is that lung sliding* is lost; the pleura are not in contact, abolishing the shimmer created by the lung surface (visceral pleura) sliding across the inside of the thoracic wall (parietal pleura). With large amounts of pleural effusion, the visceral pleura may not be readily visible; this will depend on the depth settings of the ultrasound machine (e.g. the visceral pleura may be present beyond the visible far field of the ultrasound image).

Criteria to rule out pleural effusion

There are three sonographic findings that confirm the pleura are in contact, ruling out pleural effusion (and pneumothorax) at the transducer location:

1. Complete lung sliding across the entire pleural line at the transducer location.
2. The presence of lung pathology (B lines and/or consolidation) originating at the pleural line.
3. The presence of a lung pulse.

* Recall the definition of complete lung sliding: the two pleura must be in contact, and the animal must breathe.

In addition, mirror image artifact (such as seen at the subxiphoid window with the transducer angled to observe the thorax beyond the diaphragm) rules out pleural effusion immediately below the parietal pleura at the transducer location because it is an artifact created by large differences in acoustic impedance at soft tissue-to-air interfaces (Fig. 5; video 5.6). Similarly, the detection of A lines, because they are a type of air induced mirror image artifact, also rule out pleural effusion at that transducer location.

QR
Video 5.6.
Mirror image artifact.

Criteria to rule in pleural effusion

There are two primary criteria used to identify pleural effusion:

1. There is a loss of lung sliding because the two pleura are separated by effusion.
2. The effusion is uncontained within the pleural space. As such it tends to form sharp demarcated angles and irregular borders when located in more gravity-dependent (lowest) regions, and tracks along the diaphragm (i.e. not curving around the heart). This is in contrast to fluid contained within the pericardial sac.

Note: In cases with significant pneumothorax, the presence of air in the pleural space may prevent underlying pleural effusion from being visualized. In these cases, scanning ventrally below the area of pneumothorax in a standing patient or widest part of the thorax in a lateral patient (e.g. gravity-dependent regions) may reveal the presence of concurrent pleural effusion.

Criteria to differentiate pleural from pericardial effusion

Pleural effusion can sometimes be mistaken for pericardial effusion, and vice versa, and both may be present in the same patient. Consequently, it is important to carefully assess both the pericardial and pleural spaces for the presence of fluid.

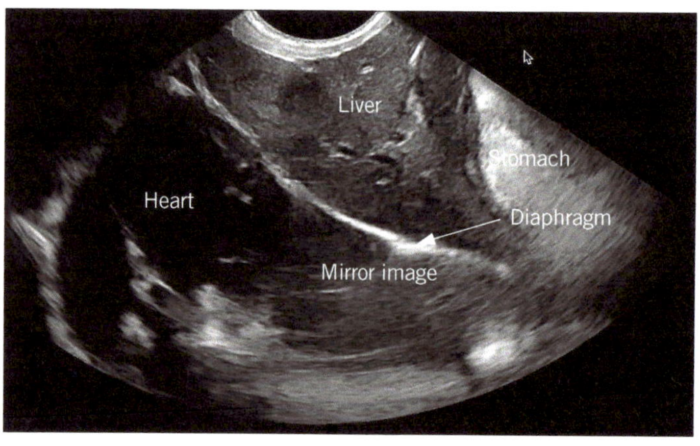

Figure 5. Mirror image artifact at the subxiphoid window, longitudinal axis.

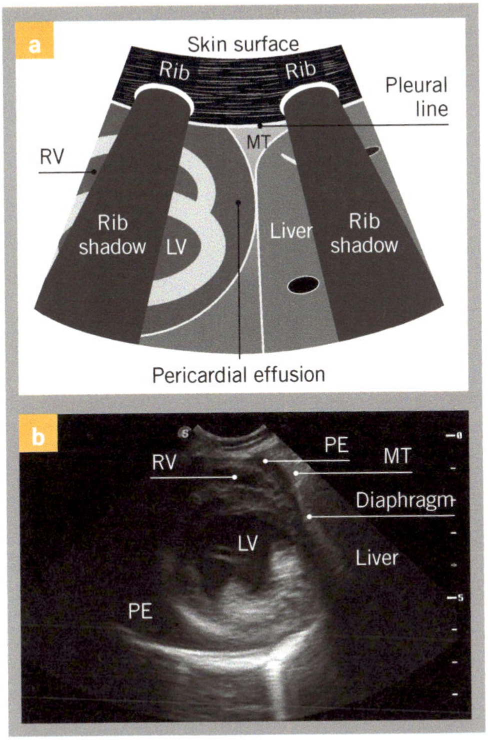

Figure 6. Schematic diagram (a) and ultrasound still image (b) at the pericardiodiaphragmatic (PD) window with the transducer in perpendicular orientation to the ribs in a dog with pericardial effusion (b). RV: right ventricle; LV: left ventricle; PE: pericardial effusion; MT: mediastinal triangle.

QR

Video 5.7. Pericardiodiaphragmatic (PD) window pericardial effusion.

QR

Video 5.8. Pericardiodiaphragmatic (PD) window pleural effusion.

Pericardiodiaphragmatic (PD) window

- At the PD window, pericardial effusion will appear as fluid contained within the pericardial sac curving around the heart and away from the diaphragm, often preserving the mediastinal triangle (Fig. 6). In contrast pleural effusion will track up and down the diaphragm, often obscuring the mediastinal triangle and permitting the diaphragm to be visible curving away from the thoracic wall, particularly when pleural effusion fills the costophrenic recess (Fig. 4; videos 5.7 and 5.8).

Right parasternal short axis views

- Becoming familiar with normal right parasternal short-axis views of the heart is key in differentiating pericardial effusion from normal cardiac chambers, such as the left and right ventricles. This will limit mistaking heart chambers for pericardial effusion. Scanning the heart from the apex, through "mushroom" and 'fish mouth" to the "Mercedes and whale" views at the heart base will also aid in identifying pericardial effusion (cardiac POCUS is beyond the scope of this Chapter).
- In the right parasternal short axis view pericardial effusion will appear as fluid contained within the pericardial sac and curving around the heart (Fig. 7a; video 5.3), whilst pleural effusion will not curve around the heart. In contrast, in healthy animals, the pericardial sac is intimately associated with the ventricular walls with no effusion separating them (Fig. 7b; video 5.9).

In both these situations, it is important to change the depth to visualize the entire heart and pericardial sac. If doubt remains as to the origin of the fluid, the transducer can be slid caudally to locate the PD window to determine if the visible effusion tracks along the diaphragm or is only contained within the pericardial sac (sometimes, both are present).

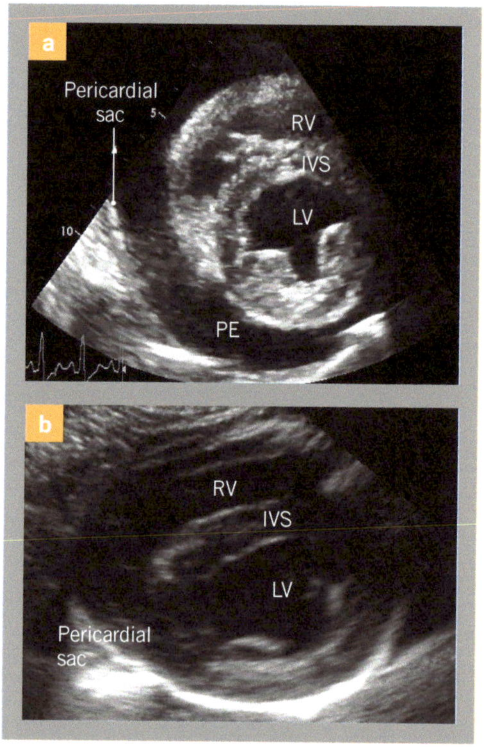

Figure 7. Ultrasound still images of the right parasternal short axis "mushroom" view in a dog with pericardial effusion (a), and a dog with a normal heart (b). RV: right ventricle; LV: left ventricle; MT: mediastinal triangle; PE: pericardial effusion; IVS: interventricular septum.

QR
Video 5.9.
Normal heart.

Subxiphoid view

Pleural and pericardial effusion can be diagnosed at the subxiphoid view in both longitudinal and transverse axis views (Fig. 8). The entire heart and pericardial sac do not need to be visualized in this window to differentiate pericardial from pleural effusion.

In most dogs and some cats, the apex of the heart contacts the diaphragm and as such the left ventricular free wall appears to blend with the diaphragm at this location (soft tissue-to-soft tissue transmission of ultrasound beams).

- If the heart is against the diaphragm with no hypoechoic fluid separating the two, then clinically significant pericardial effusion is very unlikely. The left ventricular free wall is in contact and appears to blend with the diaphragm when there is no clinically significant pericardial effusion (Fig. 8a–b; video 5.10).
- With pericardial effusion, the fluid is contained inside the pericardium and can be seen curving around the heart along the contours of the pericardial sac. The diaphragm and left ventricular free wall are separated by the pericardial effusion (Fig. 8c–d; video 5.11).
- With pleural effusion, the fluid will track along the diaphragm, and will not circle around the contours of the heart (video 5.12).

Note: in animals where the heart does not contact the diaphragm, the heart will not be visible at the subxiphoid window because lung (air) is superimposed between the diaphragm and heart, which does not transmit ultrasound beams. Cats will often have lung separating the diaphragm from the heart at the subxiphoid window.

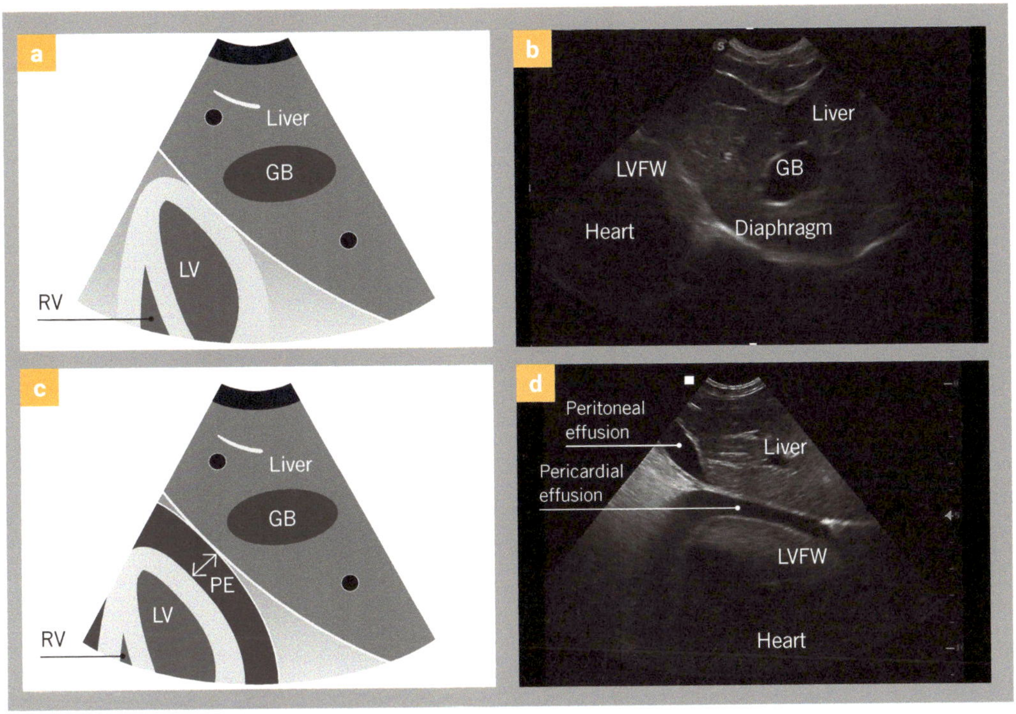

Figure 8. Schematic diagram (a) and subxiphoid long axis (ultrasound image) view (b) in a dog with a normal heart. Schematic diagram (c) and subxiphoid long axis (ultrasound image) view in a dog with a pericardial effusion (d). Note in the ultrasound image a small amount of peritoneal effusion is seen between the diaphragm and the liver. PE; pericardial effusion, LVFW; left ventricular free wall, GB; gallbladder, RV; right ventricle, LV; left ventricle.

QR
Video 5.10.
Subxiphoid cardiac blend.

QR
Video 5.11.
Subxiphoid pleural and pericardial effusion.

QR
Video 5.12.
Subxiphoid pleural effusion.

Table 1. Ruling in or out pleural effusion at the transducer location.

Rule in	Rule out
Loss of lung sliding	Complete lung sliding
Fluid tracking along the diaphragm forming angles	Lung pathology (B lines and/or consolidation) originating from the pleural line
	Lung pulse
	Mirror image artifact beyond the diaphragm or pleural line

Table 2. Ruling in or out pericardial effusion.

Transducer location	Rule in	Rule out
Pericardiodiaphragmatic (PD) window.	Effusion contained within pericardial sac encircling the heart.	No effusion present with mediastinal triangle fat most often visible. If pleural effusion: effusion outlining and tracking along the diaphragm but not encircling the heart, mediastinal triangle often replace by fluid.
Subxiphoid window.	Effusion contained within pericardial sac encircling the heart and separating the left ventricular free wall from the diaphragm.	Ventricular free wall touching and blending with the diaphragm; no separation between the two.
Parasternal (short or long axis) cardiac window.	Effusion contained within pericardial sac encircling the heart (important to correctly identify normal heart chambers).	Pericardial sac intimately associated with heart walls with no fluid separating the two (important to scan the heart from apex to base to rule out small pericardial effusions).

The shape of pleural effusion

The appearance or shape of pleural effusion varies based on its location, interaction with the heart, lungs, thoracic cage, diaphragm, presence of adhesions, quantity and the orientation of the transducer.

Perpendicular transducer orientation to the ribs:

- With small quantities of pleural fluid, fluid often appears as a hypoechoic (black) stripe, of varying thickness, separating the two pleural sheets (Fig. 1b; video 5.13).
- With larger quantities of effusion, fluid amounts may be substantial, and depth may have to be increased to visualize the visceral pleura and/or atelectatic lung.

QR
Video 5.13.
PD Deep fluid.

Parallel transducer orientation to the ribs, marker dorsally and transducer positioned ventrally (gravity-dependent region):

- When no effusion is present, the pleural line is comprised of both pleura which curves along the ventral sternal border comprised of the sternal/pectoral muscles. This image has been termed the "ski jump" sign by the authors (Fig. 9a; see video 3.13).
- When scant to small quantities of fluid accumulate between the parietal pleural lining the sternal/pectoral muscles and the visceral pleura/lung surface, the two pleural sheets will be separated, often forming hypoechoic "spinnaker sail" shaped lesions (Fig. 9b; video 5.14). Hence, the authors have termed this a "sail sign" to identify positive pleural effusion when the transducer is parallel to the ribs.
- Locating scant amounts of fluid may not have therapeutic considerations but can have important diagnostic benefits. For instance,

with a patient presenting non-specific clinical signs, finding a scant amount of pleural effusion, and possibly sampling it, may provide a diagnosis for the patient's ailment.

QR
Video 5.14.
"Sail sign".

Assessing the pericardiodiaphragmatic window and the heart via the subxiphoid window often allows pleural and pericardial effusion to easily be differentiated from each other (Fig. 2). Knowing the difference in how fluid appears at different locations is important to ensure pleural effusion is accurately identified.

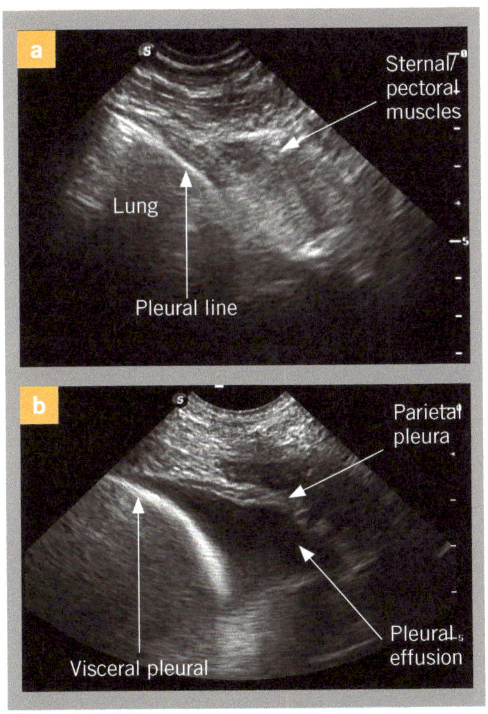

DIAGNOSTIC APPROACH

Transducer orientation and selection

A microconvex curvilinear transducer is used to search for pleural effusion. In general, the depth is set at 2–6 cm, depending on the patient's body condition score (obese patients require deeper settings, thin patients' shallower settings). To visualize the pleural line and lung sliding, a good rule of thumb is to place the pleural line at approximately the 1/3 to 1/2 mark of the ultrasound image (Fig. 10; see video 3.1).

Transducer settings are adjusted to make the pleural line appear grainy; the grainier the pleural line, the easier it is to identify lung sliding. See normal lung sliding (Chapter 3) for general tricks regarding transducer manipulation to make the pleural line grainier and lung sliding easier to visualize.

Figure 9. The "ski jump" sign; the transducer is parallel to the ribs ventrally with the transducer marker directed dorsally on the thorax in this sternal patient. The image produced when no pleural effusion is present is that of a "ski jump"; in other words, the two pleural sheets are in contact and lung sliding is seen, and the pleural line curves along the pectoral/sternal muscles (a). The "sail sign"; the transducer is parallel to the ribs with the transducer marker directed dorsally and the transducer positioned ventrally on the thorax in this sternal patient. The image produced when pleural effusion is present is that of a "sail sign"; in other words, the two pleural sheets are separated by fluid forming a triangle shape and lung sliding is absent. In a live patient, the triangle of fluid changes shape with respiration and lung expansion, giving the impression of a sail flapping in the wind (b).

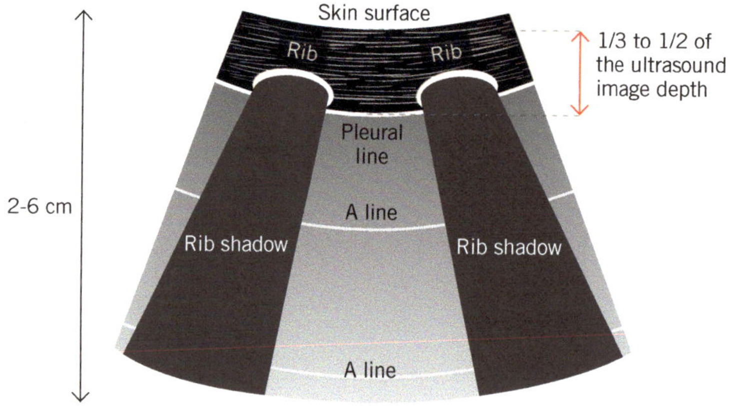

Figure 10. Schematic ultrasound image showing the recommended starting depth to initially assess the pleural line for lung sliding. The depth setting is adjusted to approximately 2–6 centimeters and the pleural line is located at approximately 1/3 to 1/2 of the depth of the ultrasound image (red arrow).

The transducer can be placed perpendicular or parallel to the ribs. The authors recommend starting with the transducer perpendicular to the ribs for beginners.

Patient Positioning

Patient positioning affects where pleural effusion accumulates in the thorax and, therefore, where it can be sonographically visualized. In standing or sternal position, fluid will accumulate in the ventral aspects of the thorax. In lateral recumbency, fluid will accumulate at the widest gravity-dependent part of the thorax. Therefore, the scanning technique should take into account the patient position (See Chapter 1; Fig. 2).

Sonographic techniques to identify pleural effusion

In general, two PLUS approaches are used to identify pleural effusion; the subxiphoid approach and the transthoracic approach.

Subxiphoid window

The subxiphoid area should be palpated and the transducer placed at this site (see Chapter 2). The transducer should be fanned and rocked in both long and short axis to increase the chance of finding smaller accumulations of pleural fluid:

- In standing position, the subxiphoid is accessed by palpating the "V" of the subxiphoid region and placing the transducer in this location.
- In sternal position, the subxiphoid region can be reached by placing two tables in an "L" fashion and laying the patient's subxiphoid region in the gap formed by the two tables, or by using a cardiac table.
- In lateral recumbency, the subxiphoid "V" can be easily reached and palpated.

The transducer needs to be more parallel relative to the spine in orientation and the depth setting adjusted (set deeper) compared to the angle and depth used for POCUS of the abdomen. This will allow the ultrasound beams to extend into the more ventral regions of the thorax using the liver as an acoustic window into the thorax.

At the subxiphoid window, pleural effusion will appear to track along (up and down) the diaphragm, forming angles (Fig. 11).

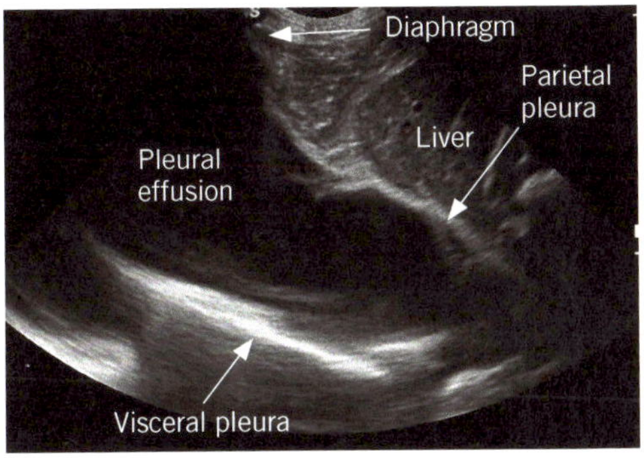

Figure 11. Pleural effusion seen from the subxiphoid view. Pleural effusion will track dorsally and ventrally along the diaphragm and the parietal pleura, outlining the diaphragm and forming angles with other structures.

Transthoracic window

Patient in lateral recumbency

Although sternal or standing is preferred when scanning the pleural space, particularly in patients with respiratory distress, some patients may require lateral positioning (e.g. fractures). The most sensitive transthoracic window to identify pleural effusion with the patient in lateral recumbency is the widest, most gravity-dependent point of the thorax (see Chapter 1). This is often the heart-base region.

- Use of a cardiac table is an easy way to access the gravity-dependent regions of the thorax.
- If a cardiac table is not available, two tables placed in an "L" shape can be used and the widest gravity-dependent portion of the thorax placed in the gap created by the "L". The transducer can then be placed in this region to identify pleural effusion.
- Alternatively, an assistant can help by gently rolling the patient into a slightly more dorsal orientation (limbs up), ensuring that the patient is not in respiratory compromise. If the patient is in respiratory distress, it should be scanned in a sternal or standing position.

Patient in sternal or standing recumbency

In sternal recumbency, the most sensitive regions to detect pleural effusion will be the ventral (gravity-dependent) portions of the thorax, including the most caudoventral thoracic border (PD window; Figs. 11 and 12), which is helpful in differentiating pleural effusion from pericardial effusion. Identifying borders (see Chapter 1), specifically the caudal (curtain) and ventral (ventral pleural border), is extremely valuable to find the region where the heart and diaphragm can be visualized in the same ultrasound image*. In brief, to reach the PD window:

- Place the transducer over lung perpendicular to the ribs and identify lung sliding. To ensure lung is scanned, initial transducer placement can be 1/3 to 2/3 the way up the thorax behind the forelimb (cranial thoracic border). When the goal is to look for pleural effusion the transducer is usually placed 1/3 of the way up the thorax. If pleural effusion is identified in this region, slide the transducer dorsally to estimate the extent of the effusion.

*Please refer to Chapter 2 for detailed technique descriptions.

- If pleural effusion is not identified, slide the transducer caudally and identify the abdominal curtain sign (caudal thoracic border).
- Once the abdominal curtain sign is identified, follow it ventrally until the heart or costochondral junction is reached. At this point the heart and diaphragm can usually be visualized in the same ultrasonographic window (PD window, see Chapter 3).
  - In healthy dogs and a few cats, the heart and diaphragm are in contact with each other and a small triangle of mediastinal fat can be visualized between them (Fig. 12).
  - In most healthy cats and a few dogs the heart may not contact the diaphragm and the mediastinal triangle is obscured by overlying lung (see Chapter 3).
  - With pleural effusion, fluid will track along the diaphragm outlining it and filling the costophrenic recess (allowing it to be seen curving away from the thoracic wall). Pleural effusion will also form angles between lung lobes and between the lung and surrounding structures. When there is significant pleural effusion present it will separate the heart from the diaphragm (Fig. 13).
- Another method to find the PD window is to identify the heart in perpendicular transducer rib orientation, and then slide the transducer caudally until the diaphragm is seen. If lung is superimposed between the heart and the diaphragm sweep the transducer ventrally along the abdominal curtain sign to try and identify the mediastinal triangle. In some patients lung will always be superimposed between the diaphragm and the heart at the PD window.
- The area cranial to the heart should also be evaluated for the presence of pleural effusion.
- At the most ventral (gravity-dependent) areas of the thorax, including the PD sites, if pleural effusion is not identified with the transducer perpendicular to the ribs, the transducer can be turned parallel to the ribs to try and identify smaller accumulations of fluid between the lung or heart and ventral body wall.
  - When the transducer is parallel to the ribs and there is no pleural effusion, the pleura will be in contact with each other and the "ski jump" sign is identified (Fig. 8a).
  - When pleural effusion is present, it will separate the pleura and the "sail sign" will be visible (Fig. 9b).
- The ventral portions of the thorax, from the caudal border (curtain) to the cranial border (thoracic inlet/forelimb), can be examined for pleural effusion with the transducer in parallel or perpendicular orientation to the ribs (see Chapter 2).
- In parallel position, the transducer can be slid a few centimeters dorsally and then back down ventrally to examine the ventral lung border for pathology as well as the ventral pleural border for pathology.

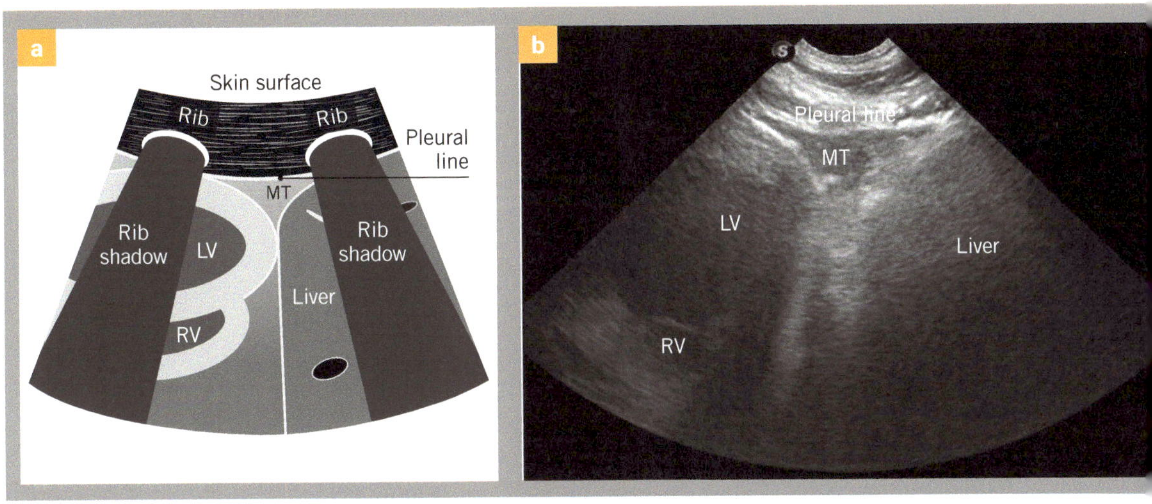

Figure 12. Schematic diagram (a) and ultrasound image (b) of the PD window with the transducer in perpendicular orientation to the ribs in a heathy cat or dog where the mediastinal triangle of fat is visible. At this window, the left ventricular free wall seen contacting the diaphragm below the mediastinal triangle of fat, because ultrasound beams travel through fat. RS; rib shadow, RV; right ventricle, LV; left ventricle, MT; mediastinal triangle.

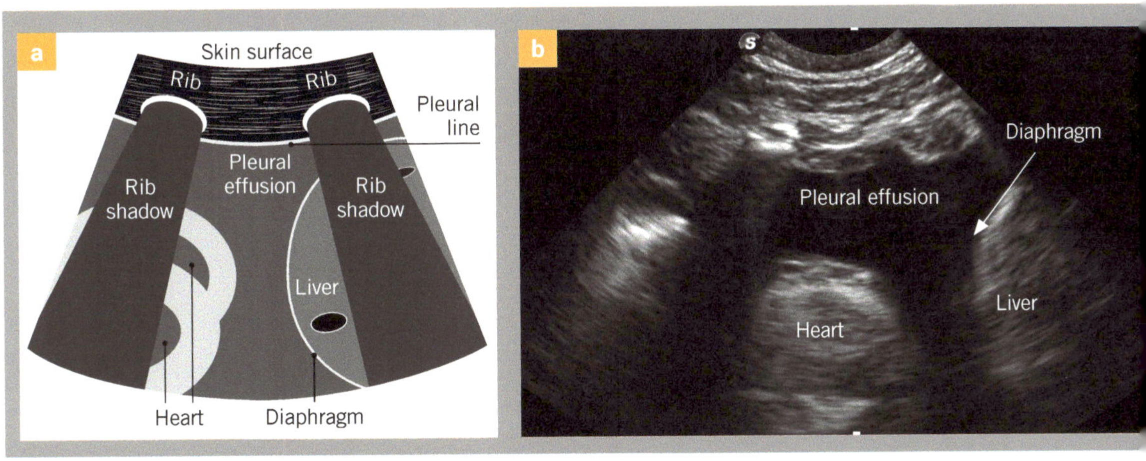

Figure 13. Schematic diagram (a) and ultrasound image (b) of the pericardiodiaphragmatic (PD) window with the transducer in perpendicular orientation to the ribs in a dog with pleural effusion. Pleural effusion tracks along the diaphragm outlining it and forms angles with other tissues/organs. The diaphragm is visible curving away from the chest wall because pleural effusion conducts ultrasound beams and fills the costophrenic recess.

BINARY QUESTIONS

In asking binary questions concerning pleural effusion, the following algorithm can be considered.

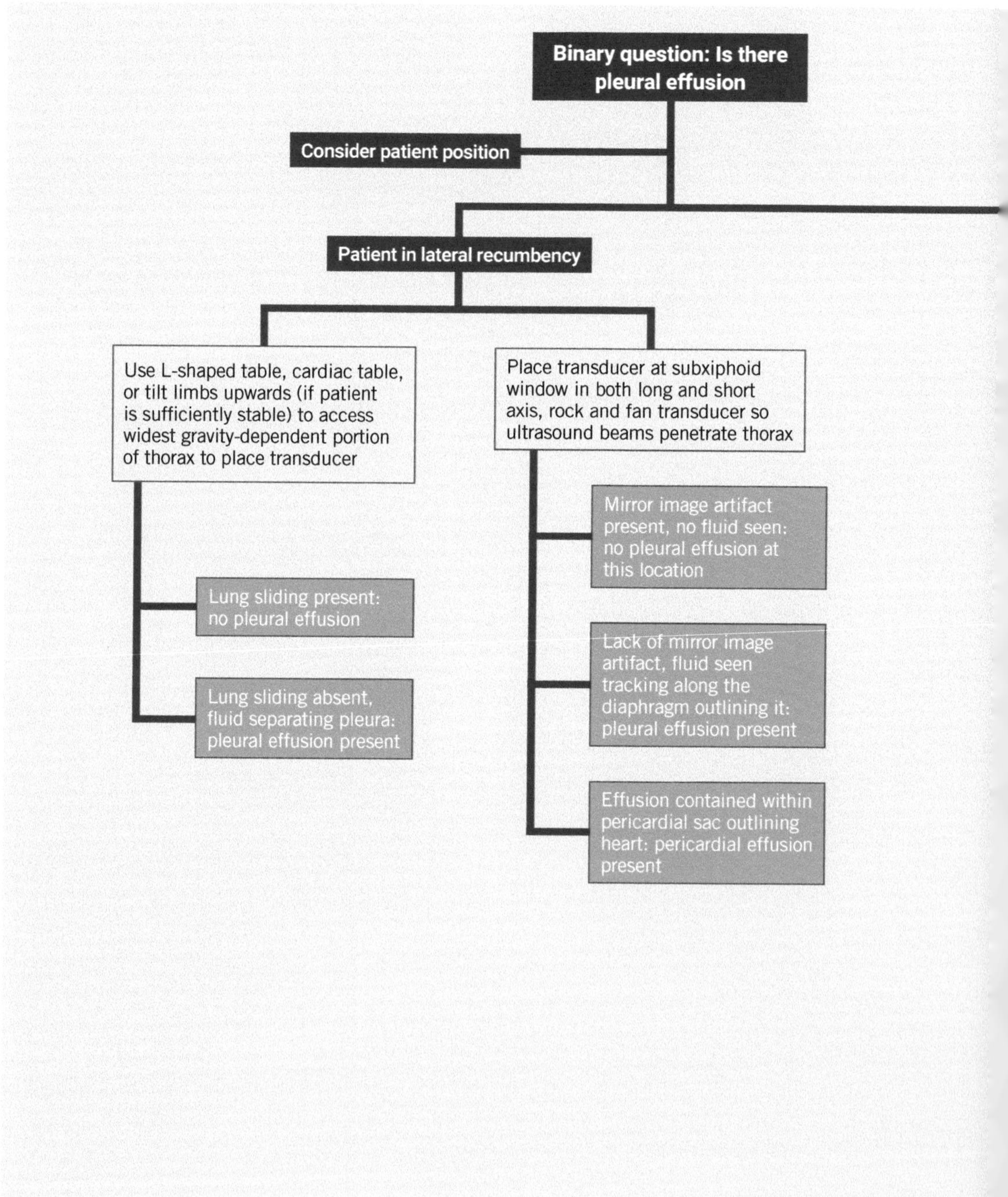

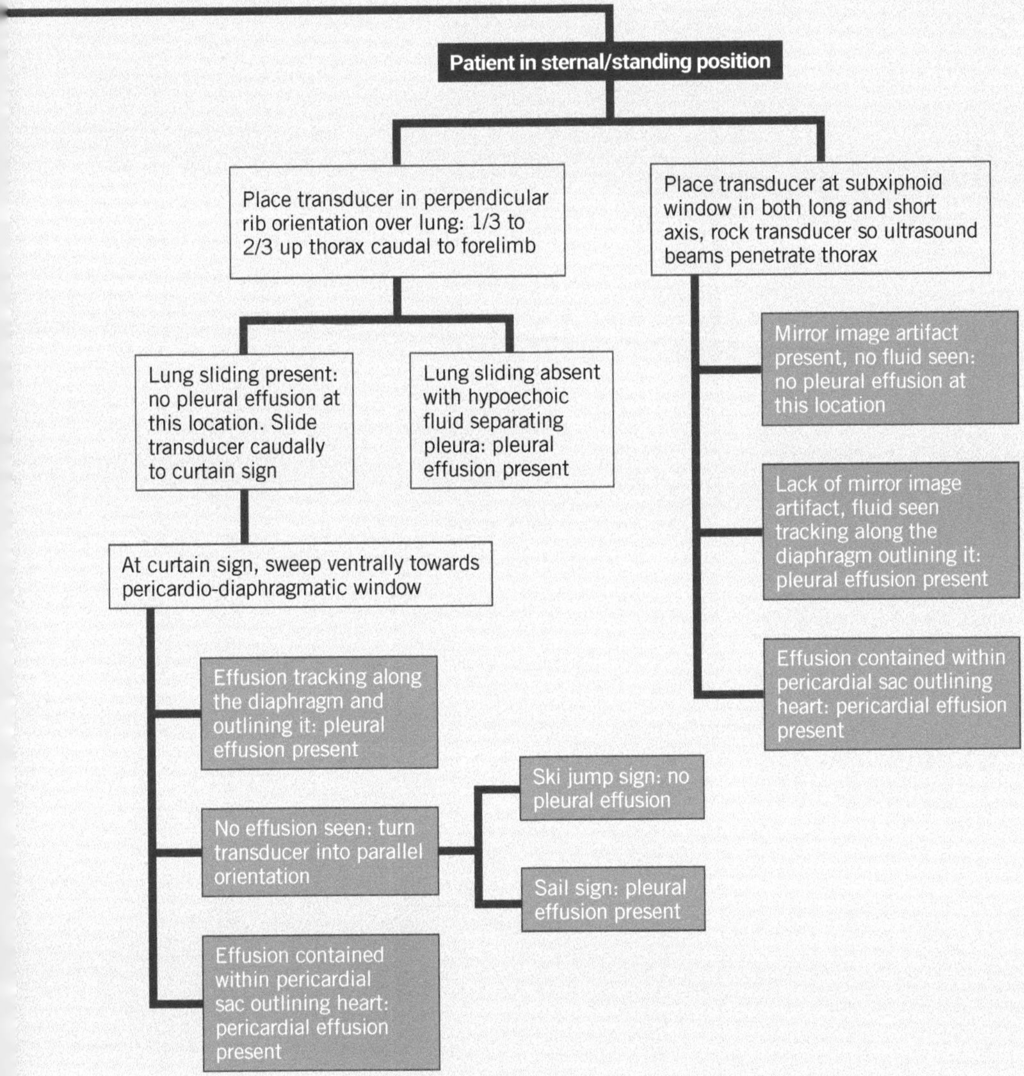
Patient in sternal/standing position
Place transducer in perpendicular rib orientation over lung: 1/3 to 2/3 up thorax caudal to forelimb
Place transducer at subxiphoid window in both long and short axis, rock transducer so ultrasound beams penetrate thorax
Lung sliding present: no pleural effusion at this location. Slide transducer caudally to curtain sign
Lung sliding absent with hypoechoic fluid separating pleura: pleural effusion present
Mirror image artifact present, no fluid seen: no pleural effusion at this location
Lack of mirror image artifact, fluid seen tracking along the diaphragm outlining it: pleural effusion present
Effusion contained within pericardial sac outlining heart: pericardial effusion present
At curtain sign, sweep ventrally towards pericardio-diaphragmatic window
Effusion tracking along the diaphragm and outlining it: pleural effusion present
No effusion seen: turn transducer into parallel orientation
Ski jump sign: no pleural effusion
Sail sign: pleural effusion present
Effusion contained within pericardial sac outlining heart: pericardial effusion present

PITFALLS

Small amounts of pleural effusion can be missed, especially if the patient presents in hypovolemia or has marked dehydration. Serial PLUS exams may help detect the accumulation of pleural effusion after restoration of normovolemia or during rehydration. Turning the transducer parallel to the ribs and scanning the most ventral regions of the patient looking for a "sail sign" in sternal may also help locate small effusions.

Pericardial effusion can sometimes be mistaken for pleural effusion, and vice versa. Assessing the PD and subxiphoid sites helps differentiate the two conditions.

Dyspneic or tachypneic patients may be difficult to image and should be scanned in sternal or standing, while oxygen therapy, anxiolytics and other stabilization efforts are employed.

SUMMARY

Scanning the thorax in a systemic fashion by finding the borders of the thorax and asking binary questions to find pathology will allow detection of pleural effusion. Large amounts of pleural effusion are readily seen and likely have therapeutic implications. Small amounts of fluid are also important to locate as they have diagnostic implications. Increasing sensitivity for finding pleural effusion can be achieved by:

- Scanning PD window in a sternal/standing patient.
- Scanning ventrally and cranial to the heart.
- Turning the transducer parallel to ribs in ventral areas of the thorax and looking for a "sail sign".
- Rocking and fanning the transducer widely and ventrally at the subxiphoid site.
- Scanning up and down the curtain sign.

REFERENCES

1. Boysen S, McMurray J, Gommeren K. Abnormal curtain signs identified with a novel lung ultrasound protocol in six dogs with pneumothorax. *Front Vet Sci.* 2019, 6:291.
2. Cole L, Pivetta M, Humm K. Diagnostic accuracy of a lung ultrasound protocol (Vet BLUE) for detection of pleural fluid, pneumothorax and lung pathology in dogs and cats. *J Small Anim Pract*, 2021, 62(3):178–186.
3. Walters AM, O'Brien MA, Selmic LE, et al. Evaluation of the agreement between focused assessment with sonography for trauma (AFAST/TFAST) and computed tomography in dogs and cats with recent trauma. *J Vet Emerg Crit Care (San Antonio)*, 2018, 28(5):429–435.
4. S. Boysen, S. Chalhoub, A. Romero. Veterinary point-of-care ultrasound transducer orientation for detection of pleural effusion in dog cadavers by novice sonographers: a pilot study. *Ultrasound J*, 2020, 12(Suppl 1): 45.

06

CLINICAL APPLICATIONS OF PLUS: ARE THERE INCREASED B LINES, YES/NO?

INTRODUCTION

Healthy lung is generally composed of air (roughly 85–95 %; predominantly within alveoli and to a lesser degree within the conducting airways), and non-aerated tissue (roughly 5–15 %; comprised of capillaries, interlobar septa, etc)[1-5]. Given that healthy lung contains mostly air, and that ultrasound beams are reflected from soft tissue-to-air interfaces, the lungs have previously been considered an insurmountable obstacle to ultrasound (Fig. 1)[4].

Abnormal lung ultrasound findings, which are a consequence of how ultrasound waves, fluid, cells and air interact with each other at the lung surface, are easily identified and interpreted, and correlate well with underlying lung pathology[4]. There are essentially two abnormal lung ultrasound findings that can be detected when scanning the lungs:

- B line artifacts.
- Lung consolidations.

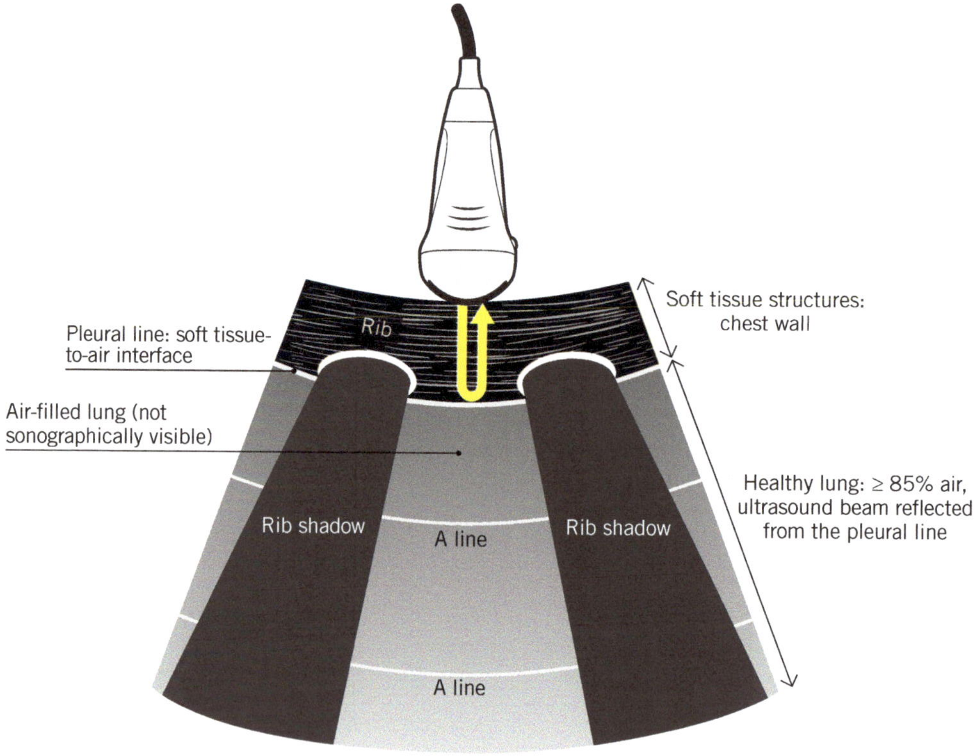

Figure 1. Schematic ultrasound image of the lungs from a healthy animal. The soft tissue-to-air interface that creates the bright white pleural line is composed of the parietal and visceral pleura. Healthy lung contains ≥ 85 % air which reflects the ultrasound beam (yellow curved arrow) from the lung surface. When the lung is in contact with the thoracic wall, the pleural line acts as a mirror to the ultrasound beam, preventing anything below it from being visualized. Although the lung is not visible, mirror image and reverberation artifact (e.g. A lines) are seen below the pleural line (see Chapter 2).

Thickened irregular pleura often occur with a progression from increased B lines to consolidation and are generally considered an early subcategory of consolidation (Fig. 2; video 6.1)[2-3].

QR
Video 6.1.
Pleural thickening.

Both B lines and consolidations share 2 common criteria that allow them to be identified:

1. They result from a decrease in the aerated/non-aerated lung ratio[1-5].
2. The decreased ratio occurs at the lung periphery, within 1–3 mm of the surface[5].

Which abnormal lung ultrasound finding is identified depends on the underlying pathology and the peripheral aerated/non-aerated lung ratio; aerated to non-aerated ratios above 10 % will reflect the ultrasound beam from the lung surface but allow B line artifacts to be detected (Fig. 3; video 6.2); when ratios fall below 5–10 % the ultrasound beam traverses lung tissue allowing lung consolidations to be detected (Chapter 7)[1-5]. Although consolidation can occur in the absence of B lines, most lung disease results in early creation of B lines as the aerated/non-aerated lung ratio falls below 85 %, with consolidations not appearing until the ratio falls below 5–10 %[1-5].

Figure 2. Algorithm depicting pleura and lung ultrasound (PLUS) findings. Abnormal lung ultrasound findings are shown at the bottom left of the algorithm, and include increased B lines, thickened irregular pleura and lung consolidations. Although thickened irregular pleura is considered a subcategory of lung consolidation, it is often overlooked and therefore should be considered separately. Abnormal pleural space findings and normal PLUS findings are shown to complete the algorithm, and reiterate how the PLUS exam is specifically designed to rapidly and accurately differentiate multiple findings using a single rapid protocol. More detail on pleural space and normal plus findings can be found in other Chapters.

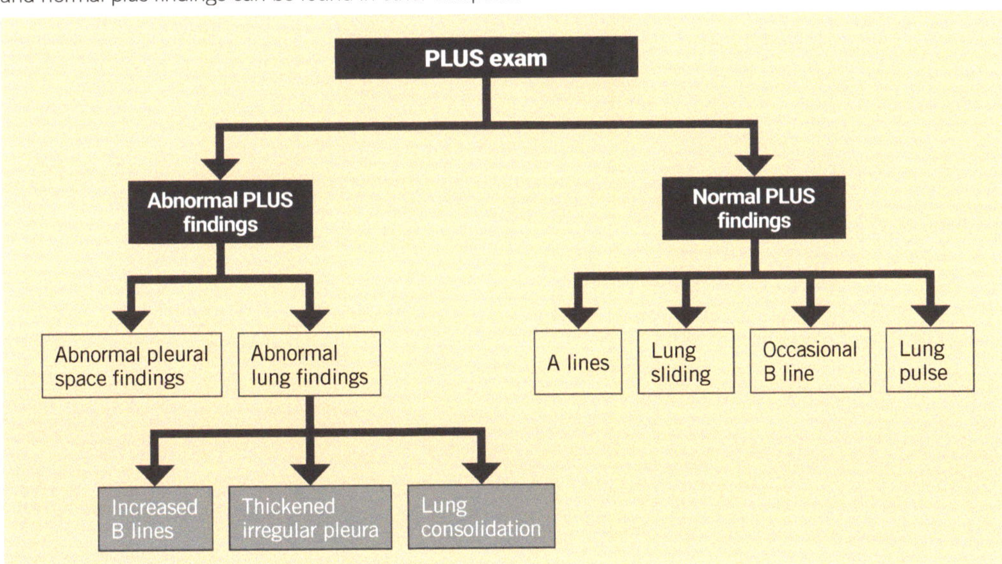

QR
Video 6.2.
Aerated to consolidated lung changes.

B lines can be an early indicator of many lung pathologies, often occurring before lung consolidations or even clinical signs occur.

The proportion of aerated lung may be decreased due to an absolute, relative or combined increase in non-aerated lung tissue. Absolute increases in non-aerated lung tissue are due to increased extravascular lung water (EVLW) or less commonly increased cell numbers (e.g. neoplasia, inflammatory cells, etc.) or tissue (e.g. fibrous tissue)[2,6]. Relative increases of non-aerated lung tissue are due to under-inflation or collapse of alveoli, as a result

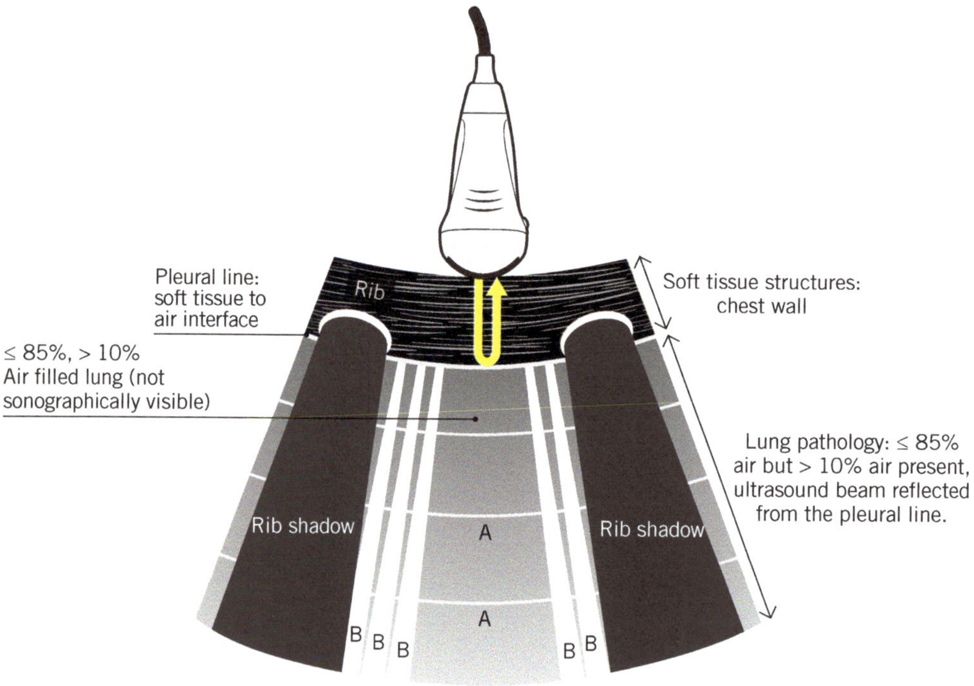

Figure 3. Schematic ultrasound image depicting B line artifacts. The lung is in contact with the thoracic wall. Although lung pathology is present below the ultrasound transducer, the lung still contains more than 10 % air in the region directly below the lung surface. Similar to healthy lung, this quantity of air in the lung is sufficient to reflect the ultrasound beam (yellow arrow) from the pleural line back to the transducer, preventing the lung itself from being visualized. However, because the lung pathology reaches the lung surface the ratio of aerated to non-aerated lung will be decreased just below the visceral pleura (below 85 %). This decrease, although not sufficient to allow the lung to be visible, is sufficient to create sonographically visible lung ultrasound artifacts arising from the pleural line (five individual B lines in this example). Therefore, even though the lung is not visible, underlying lung pathology can be diagnosed through identification and characterization of the visible lung surface B line artifacts. Research suggests that as long as ≥ 5–10 % air is present below the visceral pleura the ultrasound beam will be reflected from its surface allowing only artifacts to be interpreted. A; A line, B; B line.

of atelectasis for example. In the latter setting there is no increase in abnormal lung content but a relative increase in normal lung tissue and fluid due to a decrease of air within the alveoli (Fig. 4; video 6.3). Absolute increases in non-aerated lung tissue tend to be associated with direct lung pathology while relative increases in non-aerated lung tissue can occur in the absence of direct lung pathology (e.g. passive atelectasis)[1,2,6].

QR

Video 6.3.
Pressure atelectasis induced lung consolidation.

When B lines are the result of increased EVLW, defined as any increase in fluid within the lung, but outside the normal lung vasculature (e.g. hemorrhage, cardiogenic pulmonary edema, pus, non-cardiogenic pulmonary edema, etc.), they are referred to as "wet" B lines. In contrast, increased B lines as a result of increased cell numbers, abnormal tissue, or deflated alveoli are termed "dry" B lines (Fig. 5)[2]. Increased lung fluid and "wet" B lines are far more common than "dry" B lines, hence the term wet lung is often used when increased B lines are noted. However, as the underlying pathology and treatment is different for "wet" and "dry" B lines, identifying the cause is important[2].

Figure 4. Algorithm of absolute and relative decreases in the ratio of aerated to non-aerated lung which creates abnormal lung ultrasound findings. Relative decreases in the ratio of aerated to non-aerated lung are the result of decreased air in the alveoli creating a relative increase in non-aerated lung without an actual increase in lung fluid, cells or tissue. Absolute decreases in aerated lung are the result of an absolute increase in non-aerated lung tissue as a result of increased fluid, cells or tissue within the lung. EVLW; extravascular lung water.

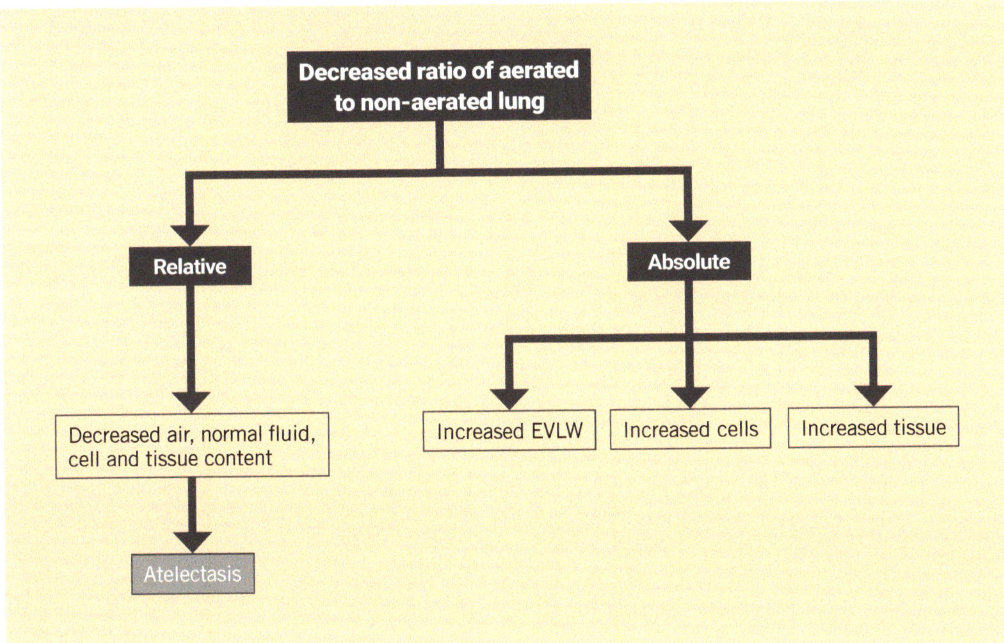

Figure 5. Algorithm for causes of increased B lines. As therapy for "dry" B lines is different than "wet" B lines, it is important to identify the underlying cause. "Wet" B-lines are caused by an increase in fluid within the lung, termed extravascular lung water (EVLW). "Dry" B lines are caused by a decrease of air within the alveoli (atelectasis) or an increase in the cell number or tissue content. EVLW; extravascular lung water, NCPE; non-cardiogenic pulmonary edema, CHF; congestive heart failure, ARDS; acute respiratory distress syndrome.

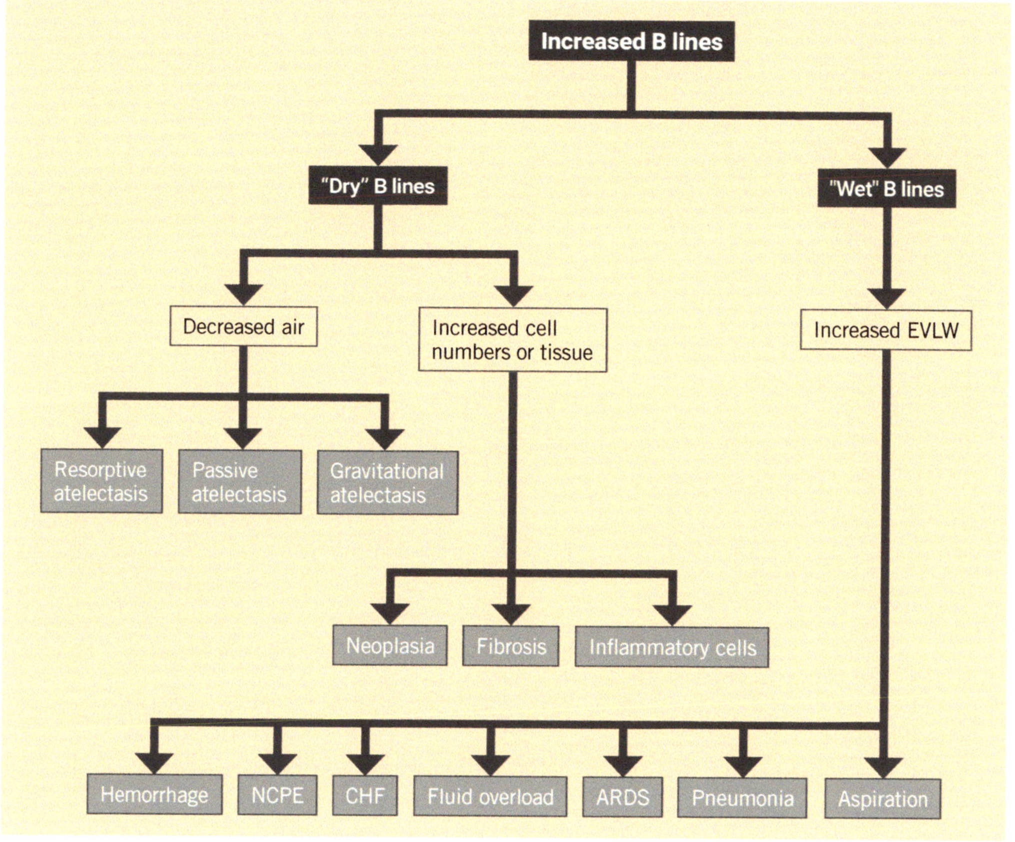

Although lung ultrasound is very sensitive at detecting the presence of B lines, the cause of increased B lines cannot be determined with lung ultrasound alone. As such, several differential diagnoses must be considered when it is detected (Fig. 5). Like thoracic radiography, which is sensitive at identifying radiographic patterns and is less specific at identifying the underlying cause, the clinician must consider the entire PLUS profile (see below), signalment, clinical examination, lesion distribution and results of other complementary diagnostics to further refine the differential diagnosis for increased B lines.

Regardless of the cause, the emphasis is on pathology at the lung periphery because pathology lying deep to the lung surface cannot be visualized if overlying aerated lung is present between the pathology and the lung surface. Fortunately, most pulmonary pathology, particularly increased EVLW, involve the lung surface to some extent, lending itself to sonographic interpretation through creation of abnormal lung ultrasound findings, particularly increased B lines[4,7]. The following chapter will discuss the ultrasonographic findings associated with the presence of increased B lines, with an emphasis on the most common causes.

Common criteria of abnormal lung ultrasound

- Abnormal lung ultrasound findings are caused by a decrease in the aerated/non-aerated lung ratio. This decreased ratio occurs within 1–3 mm of the lung surface.
- When lung tissue below the visceral pleura contains between 10–85 % air, increased B lines are seen, which correlate with underlying lung pathology.
- When ratios fall below 5–10 %, the ultrasound beam traverses lung tissue allowing lung consolidations to be detected.
- B lines resulting from increased extravascular lung water (EVLW), defined as an increase in fluid within the lung, but outside the lung vasculature (e.g. hemorrhage, cardiogenic pulmonary edema, pus, non-cardiogenic pulmonary edema, etc), are referred to as "wet" B lines.
- B lines resulting from increased cell numbers, abnormal tissue, or deflated alveoli are termed "dry" B lines.

CRITERIA TO DIAGNOSE INCREASED B LINES

Recall that occasional (1–3) B lines can be identified in up to 10 to 30 % of healthy dogs and cats, and that five criteria are used to confirm the artifact seen is a B line and not a Z or E line (Figs. 6 and 7; Chapter 2).

- Note: The term "lung rocket" has been used interchangeably with the term B line in veterinary medicine. The authors do not use the term lung rocket and prefer to use the term B line to avoid confusion; the definition of "lung rockets" is specific within human medicine and implies the presence of increased B lines (e.g. the term "lung rockets" is used when three or more B lines are present between two ribs)[3].

B lines can be identified anywhere over the lung surface; hence, it is important to scan multiple lung regions when searching for B lines. The authors recommend completing the full PLUS exam to decrease the likelihood of missing clinically significant lesions, provided the patient is sufficiently stable to tolerate the full PLUS exam. Oxygen, anxiolytics, and other therapies may improve patient stability allowing the entire PLUS and other point of care ultrasound (POCUS) assessments to be completed.

Once B lines are identified, there are two criteria used to decide if their presence is considered abnormal:

- The number occurring in a single sonographic window.
- The combined lung ultrasound findings identified over the entire hemithorax.

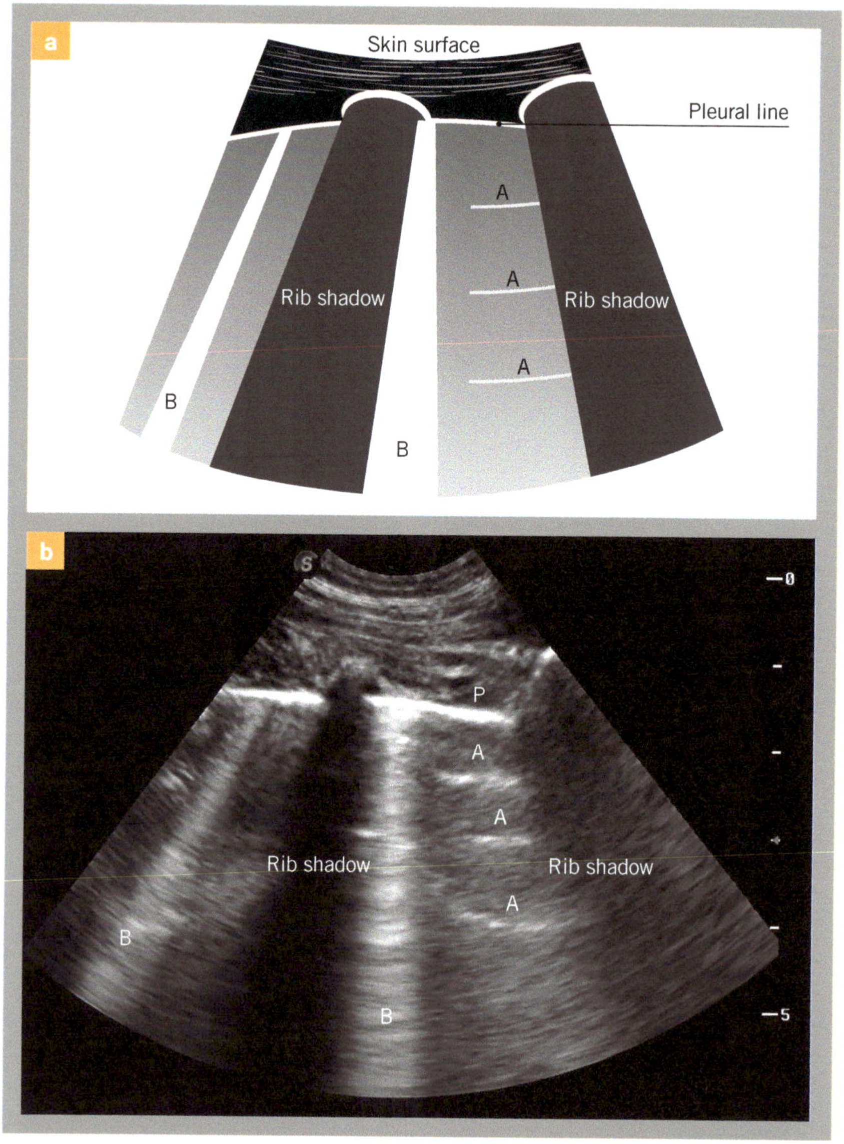

Figure 6. Schematic and still ultrasound images depicting two B lines that were identified at one location over the right hemithorax in a healthy 4-year-old DSH cat. Although there is only one B line present within each rib space, the number of B lines should be counted within the entire ultrasound image and not just between two ribs. At this single transducer location, the binary question "are B lines increased?" can be answered; however, it is extremely important not to interpret lung ultrasound findings in isolation. All lung ultrasound findings from all windows assessed over each hemithorax, and all finding from a complete PLUS exam, should be combined to create a PLUS profile for the patient. The PLUS profile must then be assessed considering history, clinical and additional point of care ultrasound findings. Only then can it be decided that the two B lines at this single transducer location are normal. Note that the width of the two B lines varies slightly in these images. They are both still considered individual B lines, as the B line to the right remains less than double the width of the B line to the left (see text). The gain in the still image should be decreased slightly to provide greater contrast between the more aerated lung and B lines. A; A line, B; B line, PL; pleural line.

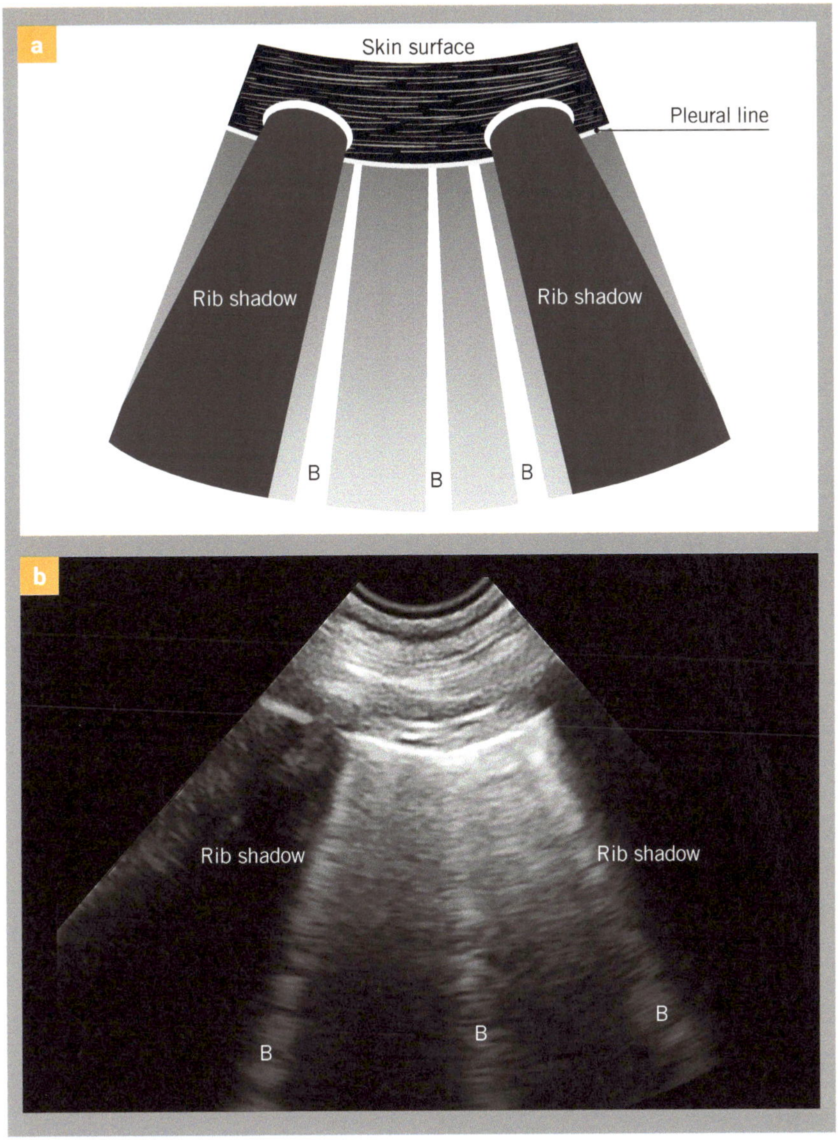

Figure 7. Schematic (a) and still (b) ultrasound images showing three single B lines identified in a 2-year-old mix breed dog. Although rare, up to three B lines in a single sonographic window can be identified in healthy dogs and cats. It is more common to find an absence of B lines, or a single/pair of B lines at only 1–2 sites over a hemithorax. The interpretation should be made considering history, clinical findings, the entire PLUS, and even serial PLUS evaluation of the patient (see text). In these images the presence of multiple individual B lines interspersed between anechoic lung creates an alternating “vertical striped” black and white lung pattern. The gain in this example has been adjusted to enhance the contrast between B lines and surrounding more anechoic aerated lung artifact, which makes the “vertical striped” lung pattern easier to see. These three B lines are of roughly equal in width making them easy to count as single B lines. B; B line.

Both questions must be answered to create an overall PLUS profile for the patient. In other words, the PLUS profile answers specific binary questions within each ultrasound window examined (e.g. are increased B lines present Y/N, is lung consolidation present, Y/N) and then combines findings from all ultrasound windows to create a "big picture" PLUS profile, which in conjunction with the history and other clinical findings, allows the most likely diagnosis to be made.

Criteria 1. Number of B lines within a single sonographic window.

Finding more than three B lines in any single sonographic window of dogs and cats is considered abnormal (Fig. 8). The width of B lines should be contemplated when counting the total number of B lines within a single window. In healthy animals, B lines may vary slightly in width and shape (Figs. 6, 7 and 8b); however, in the authors' experience, the width of the widest B line should not exceed double the width of the narrowest B line.

When pathology is present B lines may start to merge and form wider appearing B lines, often cone shaped, termed coalescent B lines

The presence of coalescent B lines makes it more difficult to determine the "true" number of B lines that are present (Figs. 8b and c; video 6.4).

QR
Video 6.4.
Increasing B lines.

Currently there is no consensus regarding when a B line that is wider than others should be considered as two or more coalescent B lines. In the authors' experience, within an acoustic window:

- Any B line that is less than double the width of the narrowest visible B line, should be considered a single B line (Fig. 6).
- If a B line appears wider than double the width of narrowest B line within the same acoustic window, particulary at its base, the authors consider this to be reflective of two coalescent B lines, or a double B line (Fig. 8b).
- Along the same lines, when a B line appears wider than three times the width of the narrowest B line it is considered to represent multiple coalescent B lines (Fig. 8b).

This is an important consideration, as a patient showing three B lines that appear wide at only one location over the hemithorax might be mistakenly considered normal if the width of the B lines is not considered (e.g. six coalescent B lines may appear as only three; Fig. 8b). In this setting, considering the history and other clinical findings, assessing the entire lung profile (scanning multiple lung regions for the presence of increased B lines and searching for other pleural and lung ultrasound abnormalities), and performing serial PLUS to assess the evolution of findings, may all assist in deciding if that specific acoustic window represents increased B lines or not. Increased B lines are often defined as > 3 B lines located between two ribs; however, the authors' use the presence of > 3 B lines within the entire sonographic window as diagnostic of increased B lines. This is based on the following considerations:

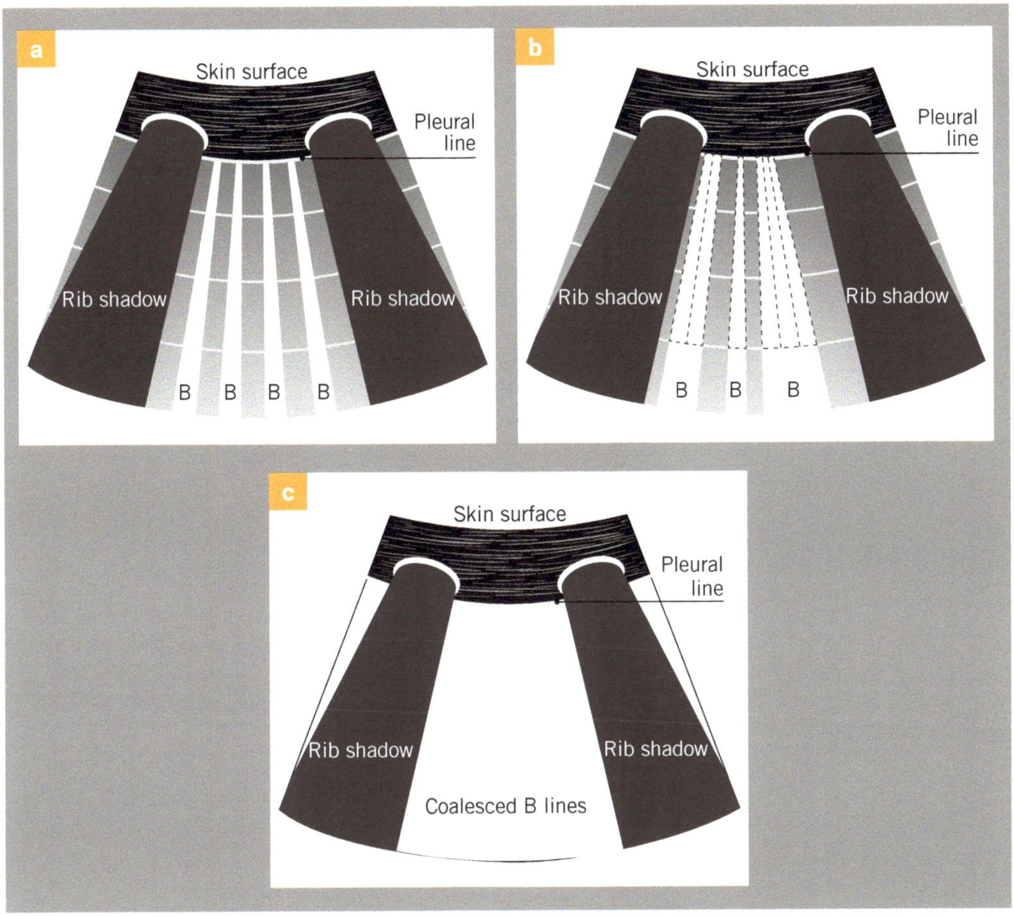

Figure 8. Schematic ultrasound images of increased B lines at three different lung ultrasound windows. Multiple individual B lines (a). When individual and separated by more anechoic lung ultrasound artifact, B lines create a "vertical striped" black and white lung pattern, making them easier to visualize. Coalescent B lines (b). Although only three vertical white lines can be counted within this schematic image, there are actually six B lines present in this image; two on the left are merging or coalescent (double B line), as are the three to the right (triple B line). The dotted lines outline the relative width of the coalescent B lines relative to the width of the single central B line (narrowest visible B line in the sonographic window). Where the pathology is significant enough, B lines completely coalesce with each other to form a solid white sheet, referred to as a "white" lung pattern (c). Note that the A lines are obliterated by "white" lung and therefore not visible in the image to the right. When "white" lung is present A lines cannot be made to appear regardless of the angle the ultrasound beam strikes the pleura. If B lines are the result of increased extravascular lung water (EVLW), the number of B lines increases as the degree of EVLW increases (e.g. more EVLW is present from left to right through the schematic images). B; B line.

- The proximity of the ribs in neonates, smaller breed dogs, and most cats.
- The movement of B lines between rib spaces with respiration.
- The fact lung ultrasound can be performed with the transducer perpendicular or parallel to the ribs, or at the subxiphoid view where ribs are not visible (Fig. 9; videos 6.5 and 6.6). Scanning the lung with the transducer parallel to the ribs allows a larger region of lung to be assessed without interference from the ribs.

QR
Video 6.5.
B lines with the transducer parallel to the ribs.

QR
Video 6.6.
Subphixoid B lines.

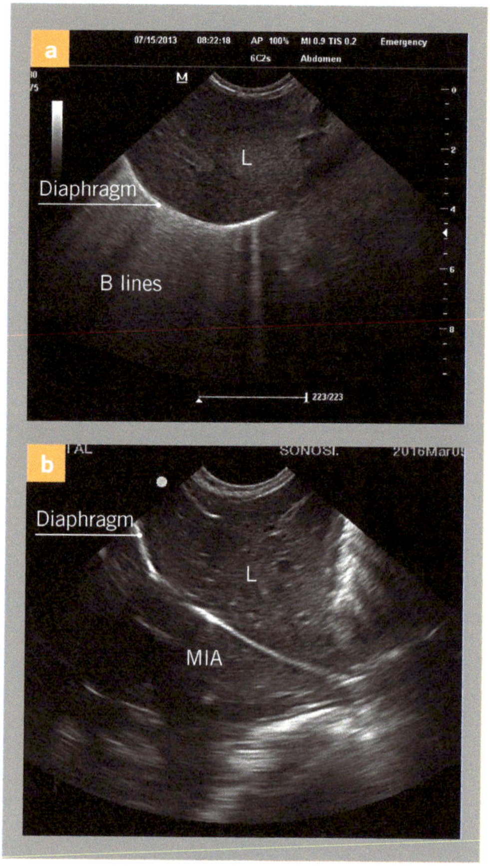

Figure 9. Ultrasound still images at the liver (near field) and thoracic cavity (far field) obtained at the subxiphoid locations. A dog with left-sided congestive heart failure showing a very large number of individual to coalescent B lines, originating from the lung surface where the lung is in contact with the diaphragm (a). Although the normal number of B lines that can be found at this location has not been reported in any species, the number visible is markedly increased and consistent with increased extravascular lung water or wet lung in this example. Image from a healthy dog with dry lung for comparison (b). Occasional B lines can be identified at this location although there are no studies reporting what the normal range should be. L; liver, MIA; mirror image artifact.

The authors use the presence of > 3 B lines within the entire sonographic window as diagnostic of increased B lines.

Further research may refine the number of B lines normally located at the subxiphoid view as this has not been well documented in dogs and cats.

Criteria 2. Identification of B lines considering the PLUS profile over the entire hemithorax of the patient

The PLUS profile is the combination/sum of all pleural and lung ultrasound findings for all individual ultrasound windows assessed during the PLUS exam. In humans, a diagnosis of increased B lines has been suggested when more than a total of five B lines are identified over a single hemithorax, regardless of the number within a single sonographic window.

The criteria used to define increased B lines over an entire hemithorax in small animals requires further research and appears to vary slightly with the lung ultrasound scanning protocol used; there is a correlation between the percentage of lung scanned and the number of positive sites with B lines in healthy animals. In general, 1 or 2 B lines, and very rarely 3, within one ultrasound window, located at only 1 or 2 locations over a single hemithorax, has been reported in otherwise healthy dogs and cats[8-11]. However a gray zone exists, and the number of B lines must be interpreted considering history and clinical findings. For example, the finding of three B lines at a single location or the presence of one B line at three locations over a single hemithorax may or may not be significant, depending on the lung ultrasound protocol used, concurrent abnormal PLUS findings, and whether B line numbers are changing over time. Consideration of the entire PLUS profile including all sites positive for B lines and other pleural and lung ultrasound findings (e.g. thickened pleura, subpleural consolidations, pleural space disease), in conjunction with the history and other clinical findings, helps determine if pathology is truly present. Serial evaluation may also be helpful as a change in the number of B lines over time suggests the ratio of aerated to non-aerated lung is changing and therefore not normal.

As underlying lung pathology progresses, B line numbers increase and will eventually coalesce. In human medicine, coalescent B lines represent more severe lung pathology compared to individual B lines, particularly when caused by increased EVLW, although this has not yet been studied in veterinary medicine (Fig. 10)[2].

As mentioned, in isolation the detection of increased B lines is not specific regarding the underlying cause. Increased B lines can be seen with atelectasis, pulmonary edema, pulmonary hemorrhage, bacterial, fungal, and viral pneumonia, aspiration, neoplasia and fibrosis; the entire PLUS profile must be considered (see Chapter 7)[1,2,6].

Prolonged positioning of patients in recumbency can result in the accumulation of gravity-dependent fluid as well as the collapsing of gravity dependent alveoli, which causes a relative decrease of air and subsequently increased B lines in those regions (see gravitational atelectasis; Chapter 7).

Two criteria to decide if B lines are increased in number

1. More than three B lines in any single sonographic window.
2. Increased number of B lines over an entire hemithorax.

To decide if B lines are abnormal, they must be considered in light of the entire PLUS profile, as well as history and other clinical findings.

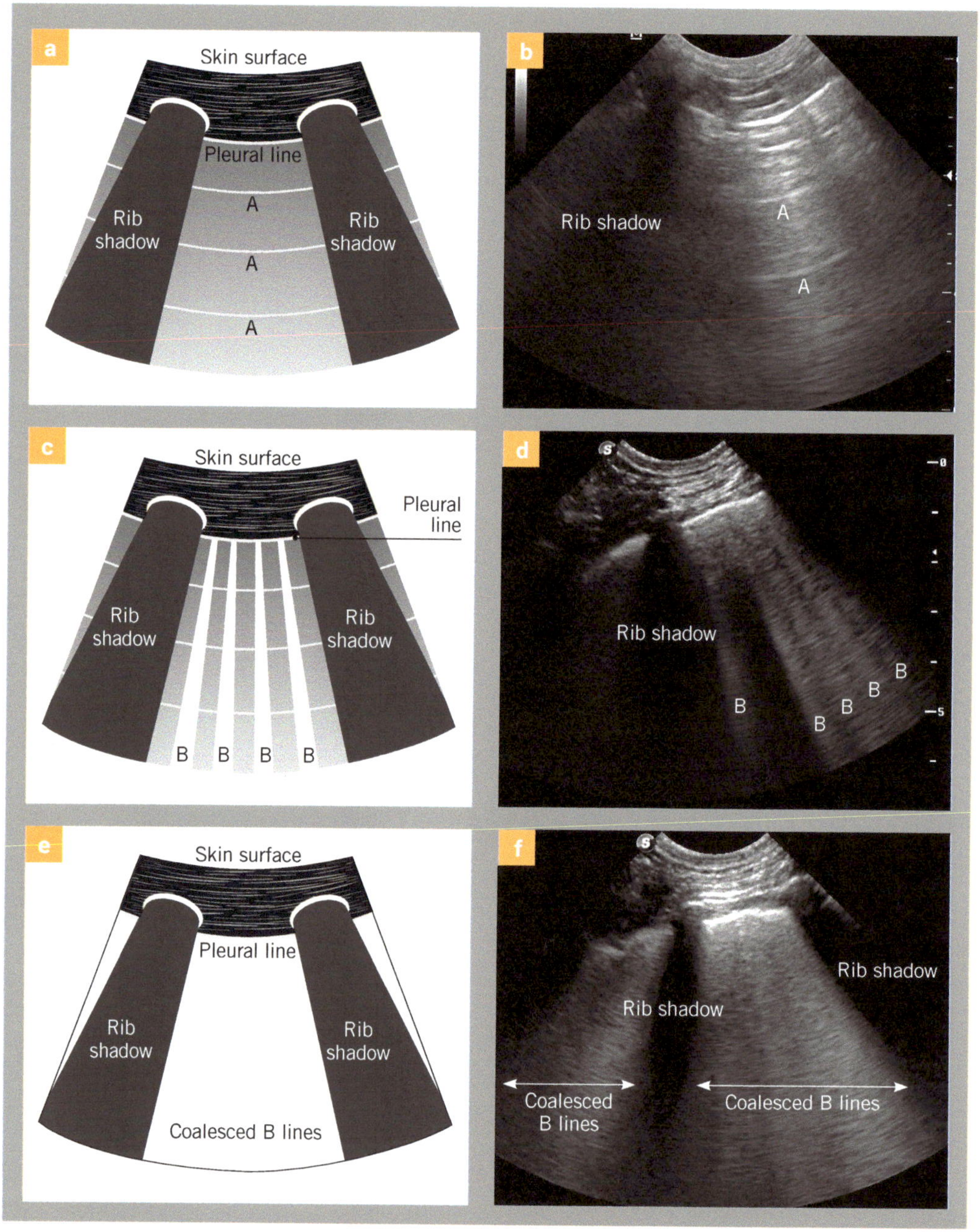

Figure 10. Schematic and still ultrasound images of dry lung progressing to wet lung with increasing extra vascular lung water (EVLW). As EVLW increases the number of B lines increases and will eventually coalesce. Schematic and still ultrasound images of dry lung (a and b). Schematic and still images of increased B lines that are still visible as separate individual B lines (c and d). Schematic and still images of coalescent B lines that are so numerous they form a solid white sheet (e and f). When EVLW is responsive to therapy (e.g. left-sided congestive heart failure and furosemide administration) the number of B lines will decrease in response to therapy as the EVLW decreases (clinical ultrasound findings move from right to left). A; A line, B; B line.

CRITERIA TO HELP IDENTIFY INCREASED B LINES

For operators less familiar with the identification of increased B lines, a few simple tricks can increase confidence in deciding if increased B lines are present:

- Machine settings, particularly the gain, can be adjusted to ensure the echogenicity of the region between the pleural line and the far field of the image is reflective of true pathology. If the gain is set to high (bright), the entire field distal to the pleural line can turn falsely "white" taking on the appearance of coalescent B lines. Use the soft tissue structures above the pleural line to properly adjust gain settings, as these soft tissue structures tend to be consistent in echogenic appearance.
- If B lines are visible against an anechoic field within the same ultrasound window, a "vertical striped" black and white pattern is generated (Fig. 11; video 6.7). The presence of a "vertical striped" pattern makes identification of B lines relatively easy as multiple single B lines, double B lines, and coalescent B lines are easily discerned if their hyperechoic cranial and caudal borders are accentuated by a more anechoic background.
- Changing the transducer angle of insonation or shifting the location of the transducer slightly on the thoracic wall may change the echogenic appearance of the B lines, creating a sharper and more recognizable "vertical striped" lung pattern.
- Assessing the far field image and extending the depth setting can be helpful in determining if B lines are present. B lines may coalesce proximally and/or distally within the image; assessing both the near and far field of the image and extending the depth may help identify a "vertical striped" lung pattern with a too and fro movement of B lines.
- Coalescent B lines, referred to as having a "white" lung pattern, may be difficult to differentiate from dry lung. "White" lung occurs when B lines coalesce to the point, they form one solid wide white sheet of B lines (Fig. 12a; video 5.4).
- With "white" lung, the entire depth from the pleural line to the far field of the image appears hyperechoic or white with an absence of A lines. It is recommended to fan the transducer when "white" lung is suspected as A lines will appear and disappear when fanning the transducer over dry lung but should always be absent when fanning the transducer over "white" lung (see A lines in Chapter 3).

QR

Video 6.7.
Black and white
striped B lines.

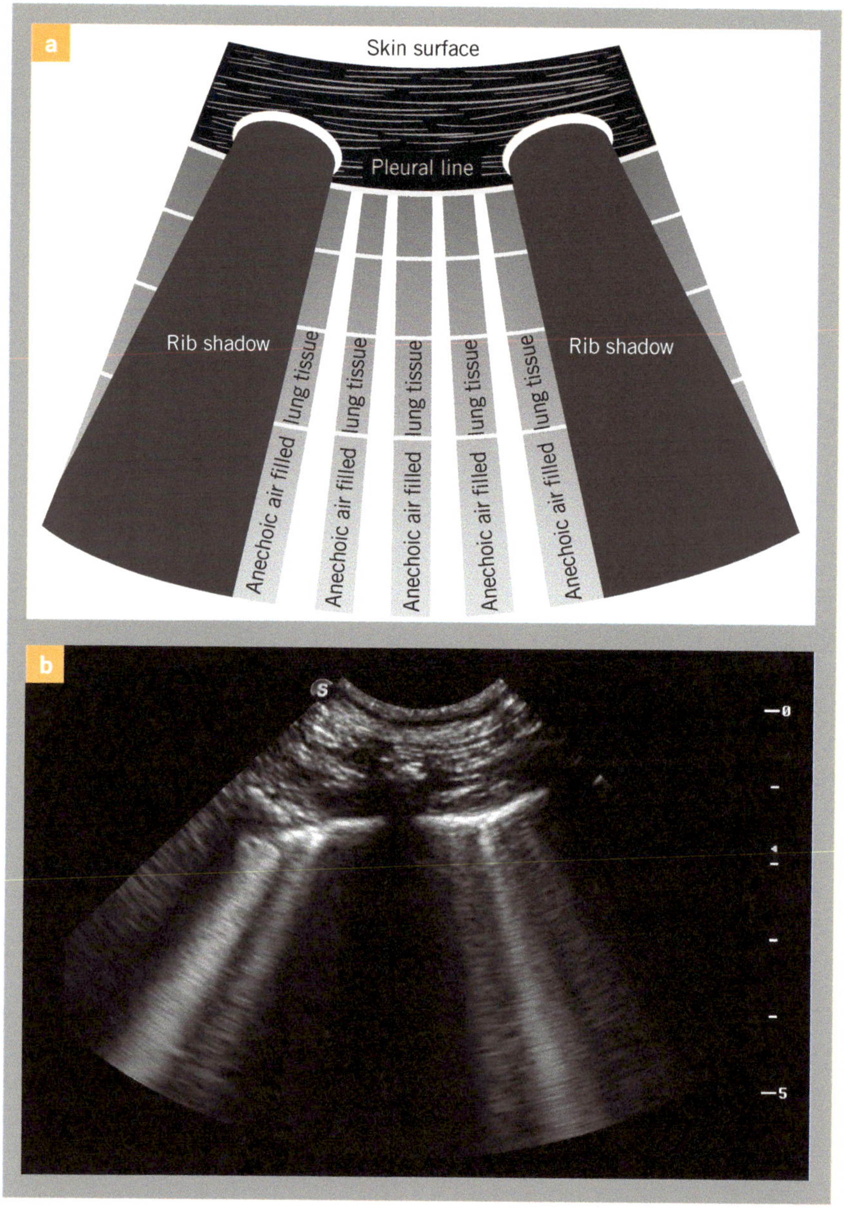

Figure 11. Schematic (a) and still (b) images of a "vertical striped" black and white lung pattern. When B lines are present within the same ultrasound window as more air-filled lung a traditional acoustic shadow (with possible A lines) will be seen, making B lines easier to identify. Sliding or sweeping the transducer from the starting location may help detect the cranial and caudal borders of B lines; defined by lung regions with a more anechoic background. Not all B lines have the same echogenicity. Changing the angle of insonation may change the echogenicity of B lines making some appear more or less echogenic.

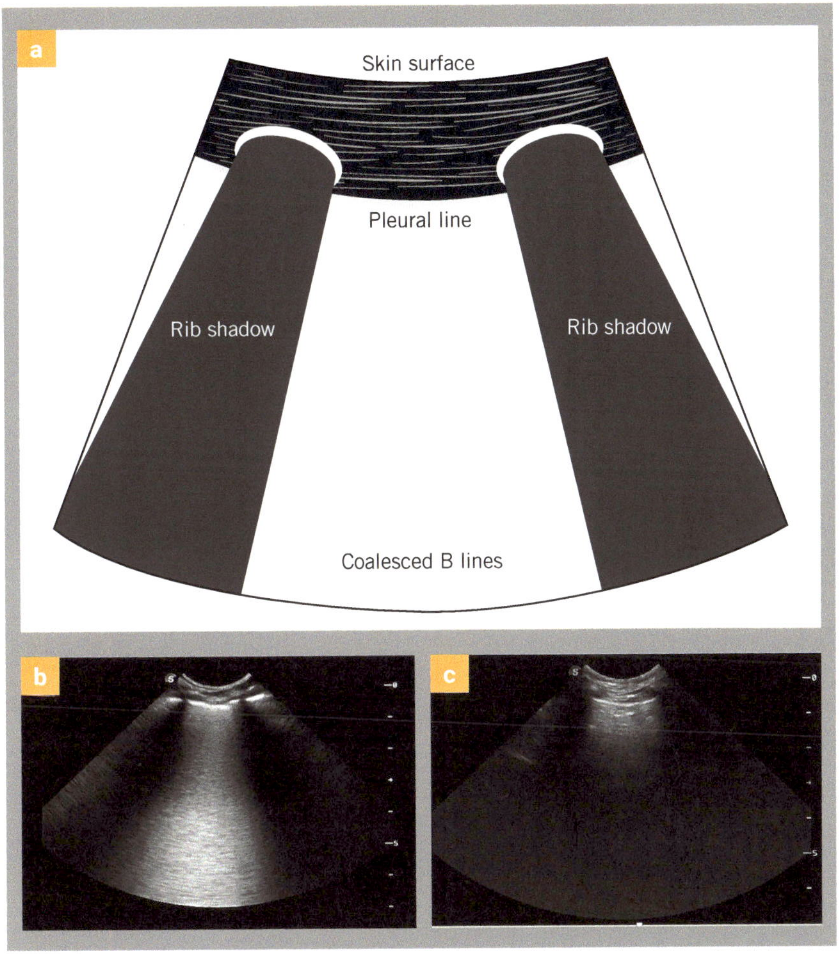

Figure 12. Schematic and still images of a "white" lung pattern (a and b) and normal lung ultrasound findings (c). With "white" lung, A lines will not be visible within the ultrasound image, regardless of transducer orientation. Fanning the transducer is recommended as A lines will appear when the transducer is held perpendicular to the pleura over dry lung, and disappear when the transducer is fanned away from its perpendicular position; they should never become visible with fanning over "white" lung (see A lines in Chapter 3). The "white" lung pattern will extend from the pleural line to the far field of the image. The pleural line is slightly thickened in the middle image, which is not uncommon with "white" lung as inflammatory lung pathology, a common cause of "white" lung, tends to create a thickened pleura (see text). In contrast the pleural line appears as a thin smooth white line with healthy lung (c). Sliding or sweeping the transducer form the starting location of "white" lung may detect a "vertical striped' black and white lung pattern if less affected lung is encountered. Alternatively, consolidation may be seen if more severely affected lung is encountered. Note that mirror image artifact is still visible below the pleural line of healthy lung, even though distinct A lines are not visible in this example. Additionally, normal lung results in a more heterogeneous echogenic appearance directly below the pleural line which tends to become more anechoic or dark within the far field in comparison to "white" lung.

- When "white" lung extends across the entire width of the ultrasound image the to and fro motion of B lines is difficult to detect as their cranial and caudal borders are not visible. Sliding or sweeping the transducer off a region of "white" lung until a different sonographic lung pattern is identified and performing a full PLUS exam allows different regions of lung to be compared and mapped. For example, "white" lung may transition to a "vertical striped" pattern if the transducer is moved to less severely affected lung or may transition to lung consolidations if the transducer is moved to more severely affected lung. Mapping the appearance and location of pathologies over different lung regions with PLUS creates a "big picture" PLUS profile, which is very helpful at determining the underlying cause.
- Finally, the appearance of the pleural line may help differentiate "white" lung from dry lung; depending on the underlying cause the pleural line may become thickened and/or develop a "moth eaten" appearance with "white" lung and will appear normal, thin, and smooth with healthy lung (Figs. 13 and 14; video 6.1)[2]. Preliminary evidence suggests the presence of thickened irregular pleura is more likely with inflammatory lung pathology such as aspiration pneumonia and acute respiratory distress syndrome and less common with non-inflammatory conditions such as left sided congestive heart failure and fluid overload; however, further research is needed to confirm these findings.

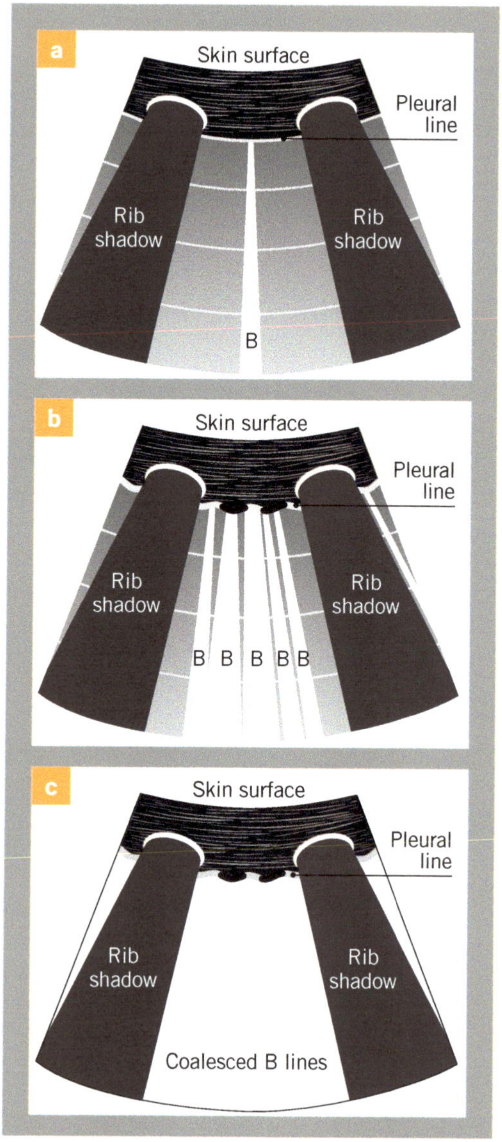

Figure 13. Schematic images of normal pleura with one B line (a), thickened irregular "moth eaten" pleura with increased B lines (b) and a thickened irregular pleural seen with "white" lung (c). Healthy lung should not have thick or irregular pleura. The presence of thickened irregular pleura in the presence of increased B lines may be more suggestive of an inflammatory process (e.g. aspiration pneumonia, acute respiratory distress syndrome, etc) as opposed to non-inflammatory causes of increased B lines such as left sided congestive heart failure or fluid overload. However, further research is required to confirm this. B; B line.

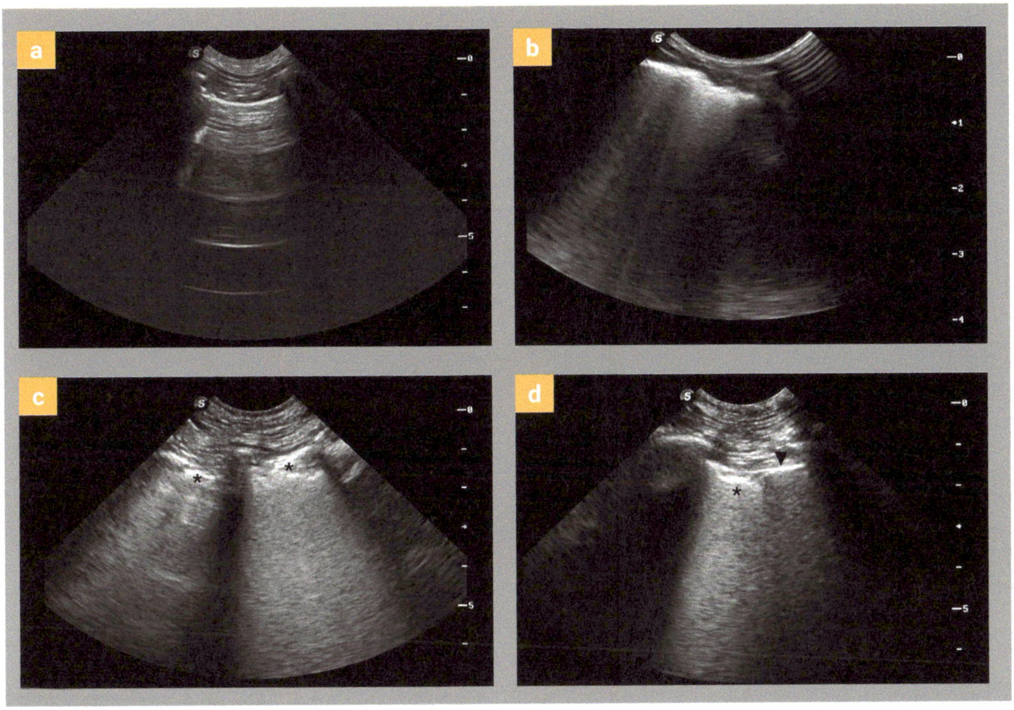

Figure 14. Ultrasound still images of normal and thickened irregular pleura. Normal lung with A lines and a thin smooth hyperechoic pleural line (a). Thickened pleural line with increased but distinct B lines (b). Thickened irregular "moth eaten" pleural line (*) with "white" lung (c). Mixed pleural line with thickened irregular lesions to the left (*) and more normal pleura to the right (arrow head) (d).

CRITERIA TO HELP IDENTIFY THE UNDERLYING CAUSE OF INCREASED B LINES

By far, the most common cause of increased B line artifact is increased EVLW, hence the reason wet lung is often used to describe the presence of increased B lines[1-5]. There are less frequent causes of increased B lines not associated with increased EVLW, such as pulmonary fibrosis (Fig. 2)[1,2]. In other words, particulate matter, cells, cellular debris, and hypocellular tissue (fibrosis, amyloidosis, etc) or even deflation of alveoli (atelectasis) can create similar appearing abnormal lung ultrasound findings to what is seen with increased EVLW.

The clinician must consider the signalment, history and clinical findings as well as the PLUS profile to differentiate if B lines are "wet" or "dry" in origin.

Whether B lines develop acutely or chronically can help determine the most likely cause in some cases:

- The acute appearance of B lines is most often associated with increased EVLW or wet lung[2]. In contrast, chronic diseases such as pulmonary fibrosis, interstitial lung disease, and longstanding pulmonary infections may lead to dilated septa, decreased aerated lung, and creation of B line artifacts with minimal increase in EVLW. As mentioned, the latter causes have sometimes been referred to as "dry" B lines to differentiate them from "wet" B lines.
- Tracking changes in the number of B lines over time in response to therapy may help decide if B lines are "wet" or "dry"[2]. In general, "dry" B lines tend to be more resistant and slower to respond to therapy vs. "wet" B lines, which tend to resolve more acutely in response to successful therapy. For example:
    - "Wet" B lines associated with left-sided congestive heart failure correlate well with resolution of pulmonary edema following a positive response to furosemide administration.
    - In contrast, "dry" B lines as a result of fibrosis tend to persist regardless of therapy.

  However, it must be emphasized that considerable overlap exists and the persistence or progression of B lines should prompt consideration of both a failure to respond in the face of a correct diagnosis for increased B lines, and the possibility of a different cause for increased B lines than initially suspected.
- The appearance of the pleural line may help determine the underlying cause. In people, a thickened pleural line is believed to occur as a result of inherent pulmonary disease (e.g. pneumonia, contusions, inflammatory lung diseases), while a thin smooth pleural line is more consistent with non-inflammatory causes of increased B lines such as cardiogenic pulmonary edema and/or volume overload (Figs. 13 and 14)[2]. This has not received much attention in veterinary medicine, although research is ongoing.
- Finally, mapping the lung ultrasound findings over the hemithorax by answering binary questions at each window (consolidation and/or B lines present: Y/N), and then combining the findings is very helpful to determine the underlying cause. For example, sliding off an area of increased B lines in the mid-thoracic perihilar region onto an area of lung consolidation in the cranioventral region is suggestive of aspiration pneumonia, particularly if supported with other clinical findings such as a history of acute onset of respiratory distress following an episode of vomiting. In contrast, the finding of diffuse B lines in three or more lung regions on both sides of the thorax interspersed with spared lung regions, with or without regions of consolidation and pleural thickening is more suggestive of acute respiratory distress syndrome (ARDS). Left sided congestive heart failure tends to cause diffuse bilateral B lines over multiple lung regions in the absence of consolidation and pleural line thickening. The history, clinical findings and assessing the left atrial size with POCUS will help differentiate ARDS from left sided congestive heart failure.

Key concepts

- PLUS allows for easy recognition of abnormal B lines, decreasing the risk for the patient.
- Increased B lines are diagnosed by identifying more than three B lines and/or coalescent B lines in a single window and considering their presence in light of the entire PLUS profile.
- The number of B lines is correlated with the amount of fluid in the lung when caused by increased extravascular lung water.
- Increased B lines can be found at any sonographically visible region of the lung surface.
- Performing a full PLUS exam decreases the likelihood of missing significant abnormalities.
- Signalment, history, clinical examination findings, results of complementary examinations as well as the PLUS profile can help refine the diagnosis.

CRITERIA TO RULE OUT INCREASED B LINES

Identifying dry lung (see Chapter 3) rules out the presence of "wet" B lines at the transducer location. As lung ultrasound only detects peripheral lung pathology, diseases failing to reach the lung surface will remain undetected. However, as mentioned, most pathology that causes increased B lines are the result of increased EVLW, which typically reach the lung surface. Therefore, detecting the presence of lung sliding in the absence of B lines makes pathologies that cause "wet" B lines below the transducer location very unlikely. As B lines can be regional, the entire lung profile must also be considered before deciding the lung is truly dry over the entire hemithorax.

Table 1. Ruling in or out increased B lines at the transducer location.

Rule in	Rule out	Do NOT assess region UNDER	Cannot assess if
> 3 B lines	Dry lung	Pleural effusion	Pneumothorax or significant subcutaneous emphysema is present
Coalescent B lines		Lung consolidations	

DIAGNOSTIC CONSIDERATIONS FOR SPECIFIC CAUSES OF INCREASED B LINES

Once increased B lines have been confirmed, their interpretation is dependent on history, clinical findings and creating the entire PLUS profile (see Chapter 7), which is combined with other POCUS findings (including abdominal and cardiovascular POCUS), to arrive at a diagnosis.

In human medicine, multiple lung ultrasound protocols have been incorporated into algorithms to help guide therapy and diagnosis (e.g. SESAME protocol in cardiac arrest and resuscitation, FALLS protocol for cardiovascular collapse, and BLUE protocols). Similar algorithms and protocols have not yet been established in veterinary medicine. However, the authors believe that by performing a complete PLUS exam, assessing the specific PLUS profile for each patient, and by integrating other clinical findings, the operator will be able to identify most abnormal lung findings and the associated underlying pathology. It should be noted that except for congestive heart failure, aspiration pneumonia and traumatic pulmonary contusions, the lung ultrasound profiles associated with underlying pathology in veterinary medicine are not well established and further research is needed to further define small animal PLUS profiles. However, the authors' current expert consensus on the most likely distributions of increased B lines and associated underlying pathology are presented in Table 2. Regardless of the appearance and distribution of increased B lines, findings should always be interpreted considering all clinical findings. As mentioned previously, false negative results may occur if lesions do not reach the lung periphery.

Although research is lacking, the use of serial lung ultrasound scanning is recommended to track progression or resolution of abnormal PLUS findings, including the number of B lines. Evidence supports a direct correlation between the number and severity of B lines and severity of EVLW with left-sided congestive heart failure; B lines decrease in number as patients respond to furosemide administration and have been used to help guide furosemide requirements. Conversely serial PLUS is sensitive at detecting the development of and/or an increase in the number of B lines in cases that develop pulmonary edema (volume overload) following fluid therapy. Serial PLUS plays an important role as an early detector of volume overload in patients receiving IV fluid therapy. Similar to all PLUS exams, assessment of other POCUS findings (e.g. left atrial size, caudal vena cava size and change with the respiratory cycle), history and clinical findings will help determine the reason for increasing or decreasing B lines when followed serially.

Patient positioning

B lines can be identified in any lung field, regardless of patient positioning. The authors therefore recommend performing the full PLUS exam in the position the patient is most comfortable, particularly if they are in respiratory distress; this often equates to the patient being in sternal recumbency or a standing position. When the patient presents and appears comfortable in lateral recumbency, repositioning the patient is not required to

Table 2. Lung ultrasound B line distribution and most likely associated causes.

Symmetrical	Asymmetric
■ Diffuse; bilateral: ■ Causes of increased hydrostatic pressure: ■ Left sided congestive heart failure (LCHF). Note that the absence of increased B lines in a dyspneic patient essentially rules out LCHF. ■ Volume overload. ■ The presence of thickened pleura and lung ultrasound consolidations are usually absent.	■ Regional: ■ Focal, anywhere: neoplasia, pulmonary thromboembolism*. ■ Right middle to cranial ventral: aspiration pneumonia. ■ Ventral, lobar: pulmonary hemorrhage, aspiration, neoplasia. ■ Thickened pleura and lung ultrasound consolidations often present.
■ Regional; bilateral: ■ Causes of caudodorsal, non-cardiogenic pulmonary edema: ■ Upper airway obstruction, e.g. choke. ■ Electrocution. ■ Neurogenic conditions. ■ Smoke inhalation. ■ Thickened pleura and lung ultrasound consolidations may be present.	■ Unilateral: ■ Trauma, pulmonary contusions. ■ Thickened pleura and lung ultrasound consolidations often present.

* *Pulmonary thromboembolism*: Although not well documented in veterinary medicine, in the authors experience pulmonary thromboembolism can also be associated with the appearance of increased B lines in dogs. In human medicine pulmonary thromboembolism is typically associated with wedge shaped lung consolidations as well as with deep vein thrombosis (see Chapter 7). The architecture of the pulmonary vasculature however varies tremendously between species, which likely explains the likelihood of finding B lines in dogs.

* *Note*: Feline asthma has not been well studied. In humans the detection of B lines with asthma is rare, and the absence of lung ultrasound findings in dyspneic casts should prompt consideration of feline asthma. However, the authors have identified increased B lines and even lung consolidation in some cats with confirmed asthma in the absence of congestive heart failure and other lung pathology. The finding of increased B lines and consolidation in feline asthma would not be surprising given a fair number of feline asthma cases have right middle lung lobe consolidation on radiographs. Further research is needed to determine the PLUS profile of cats with asthma.

perform a PLUS exam. However, prolonged recumbency can result in gravity dependent atelectasis in the gravity dependent lung lobes and the creation of B lines and lung consolidation (see Chapter 7). If abnormal ultrasound findings are identified in the gravity dependent lung lobes of a patient that experiences prolonged lateral recumbency, it is advised to repeat the PLUS exam following patient repositioning, provided it is safe to do so. If possible, walking the patient and/or maintaining the patient in sternal recumbency is preferred if the patient is sufficiently stable.

PITFALLS

- B lines can only be detected if they reach the lung surface; smaller and centrally located lesions remain undetected.
- An increased number of B lines does not discern the underlying cause or type of fluid in the cases of increased EVLW. The history and other clinical findings, as well as PLUS profile (distribution of B lines in conjunction with other PLUS findings (consolidation, irregular pleura, etc), and other POCUS findings (e.g. left atrial enlargement) should all be considered to arrive at a diagnosis.
- Coalescent B lines can be harder to identify if the clinician is unfamiliar with machine settings, fails to compare images between different windows, or fails to identify A lines within the image.
- If pneumothorax is present (absent lung sliding) at the transducer location, the lung cannot be assessed, as it is separated from the thoracic wall by a layer of air that blocks the ultrasound beam from reaching it.
- If pleural effusion is present (fluid separating the parietal and visceral pleura), abnormal ultrasound lung findings, including B lines, should be interpreted with caution as passive atelectasis secondary to pleural effusion will create artifact that is not easy to distinguish from true lung pathology. Re-evaluation of the lung following removal of pleural fluid and serial monitoring for resolution or progression of persistent abnormal lung ultrasound findings is recommended.
- Rib shadows can interfere with interpretation of lung ultrasound or hide local pathology if it is hidden below rib shadows. Identification of the "bat sign" (see Chapter 3) and turning the transducer parallel to the ribs should help uncover hidden pathology.
- B lines originating from the pleural line to either side of consolidated lung should be interpreted. However, ring down artifact (which strongly resembles B lines) originating from the distal border of partial lung lobe consolidations (not the pleural line) should not be overinterpreted as their diagnostic utility to detect and interpret lung pathology has not been investigated (see Chapter 7).

APPLICATION OF PLUS ALGORITHM

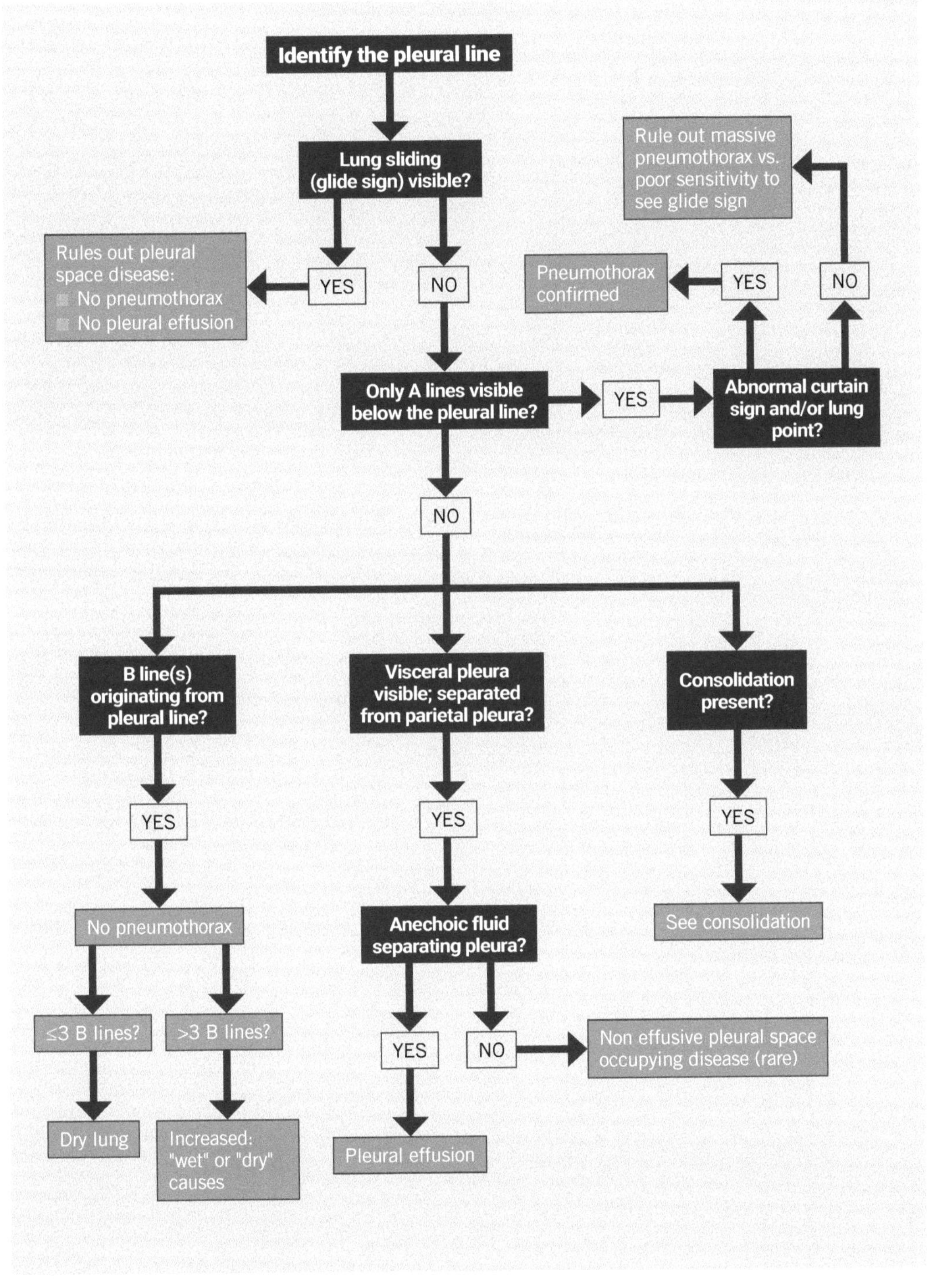

SUMMARY

Abnormal lung ultrasound findings, including increased B lines, are the results of a decrease in the ratio of aerated to non-aerated lung tissue occurring in proximity to the lung surface. An increase in the proportion of non-aerated lung may be absolute or in the case of atelectasis, relative. An increase in EVLW is the most common cause for an absolute increase in non-aerated lung and increased B lines, referred to as wet lung. The number of B lines is proportional to the severity of lesions, and in the case of wet lung correlates with the degree of EVLW. Performing a full PLUS exam and mapping the distribution of B lines through creation of a PLUS profile allows lung regions to be categorized as wet or dry at each transducer location and helps determine the underlying cause. The PLUS profile can help the clinician refine the differential diagnosis; however, it is important to consider the entire clinical picture and results of other complementary diagnostic tests, including other POCUS findings.

REFERENCES

1. Miller A. Practical approach to lung ultrasound. *BJA Education*, 2016, 16(2):39–45.
2. Picano E, Pellikka PA. Ultrasound of extravascular lung water: a new standard for pulmonary congestion. *Eur Heart J.* 2016, 37(27):2097–2104.
3. Lichtenstein DA. Current misconceptions in lung ultrasound: a short guide for experts. *Chest*, 2019,156(1):21–25.
4. Lichtenstein DA, Mezière GA. Relevance of lung ultrasound in the diagnosis of acute respiratory failure: the BLUE protocol. *Chest*, 2008, 134(1):117–125.
5. Soldati G, Sher S, Testa A. Lung and ultrasound: time to "reflect". *Eur Rev Med Pharmacol Sci*, 2011, 15(2):223–227.
6. Cereda M, Xin Y, Goffi A, et al. Imaging the Injured Lung: Mechanisms of Action and Clinical Use [published correction appears in *Anesthesiology.* 2019 Aug;131(2):451]. *Anesthesiology.* 2019, 131(3):716–749.
7. Lichtenstein DA, Lascols N, Meziere G, Gepner A. Ultrasound diagnosis of alveolar consolidation in the critically ill. *Intensive Care Med*, 2004, 30: 276–281.
8. Lisciandro GR, Fosgate GT, Fulton RM. Frequency and number of ultrasound lung rockets (B-lines) using a regionally based lung ultrasound examination named vet BLUE (veterinary bedside lung ultrasound exam) in dogs with radiographically normal lung findings. *Vet Radiol Ultrasound*, 2014, 55(3):315–322.
9. Rademacher N, Pariaut R, Pate J, et al. Transthoracic lung ultrasound in normal dogs and dogs with cardiogenic pulmonary edema: a pilot study. *Vet Radiol Ultrasound*, 2014, 55(4):447–452.
10. Vezzosi T, Mannucci T, Pistoresi A, et al. Assessment of Lung Ultrasound B-Lines in Dogs with Different Stages of Chronic Valvular Heart Disease. *J Vet Intern Med*, 2017, 31(3):700-704.
11. Lisciandro GR, Fulton RM, Fosgate GT, Mann KA. Frequency and number of B-lines using a regionally based lung ultrasound examination in cats with radiographically normal lungs compared to cats with left-sided congestive heart failure. *J Vel Emerg Crit Care*, 2017, 27(5):499–505.

07

CLINICAL APPLICATIONS OF PLUS: IS THERE LUNG CONSOLIDATION, YES/NO?

INTRODUCTION

Healthy lung is comprised of roughly 85–95 % air and only about 5–15 % non-aerated tissue[1-5]. A change in the ratio of aerated to non-aerated lung within 1–3 mm of the lung surface results in specific abnormal lung ultrasound findings, mainly increased B lines and lung consolidation (Fig. 1).

As long as there is sufficient air within the lung tissue directly below the visceral pleura, the soft tissue-to-air interface at the pleural line is maintained and the ultrasound beam is reflected, rendering the lung invisible (Figs. 2a and b)[2]. In this setting, it is only possible to visualize lung pathology though interpretation of lung surface artifact such as increased B lines (Fig. 2b; Chapter 6)[1-5].

Figure 1. Lung ultrasound findings with different ratios of aerated to non-aerated lung just below the lung surface. The left side of the algorithm shows normal findings when the ratio of aerated to non-aerated lung is > 85 %. The right side of the algorithm shows abnormal lung ultrasound findings that occur when the ratio of aerated to non-aerated lung falls below a certain percentage (< 85 % in this example). The decrease in the ratio of aerated to non-aerated lung can be due to any combination of increased extravascular lung water, increased tissue content (e.g. fibrosis), increased cell numbers (e.g. neoplasia), or due to a decrease of air within the alveoli/airways (e.g. atelectasis). If the ratio remains above 10 % then only lung ultrasound surface artifact is seen (e.g. increased B lines). When the ratio falls below 5–10 % the lung itself contains so little air that it becomes sonographically visible as consolidation. EVLW; extra vascular lung water.

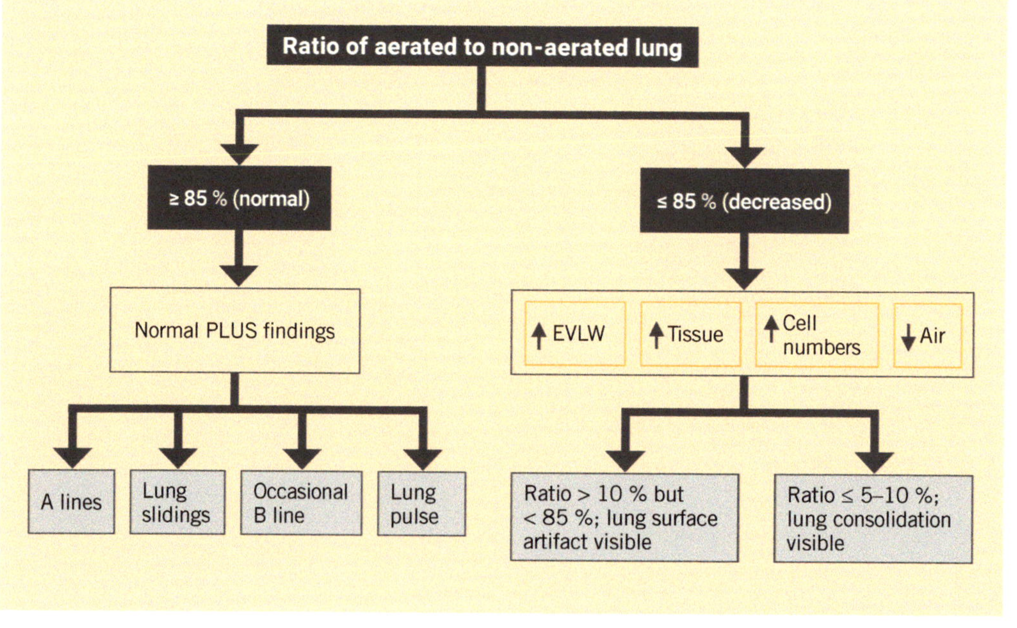

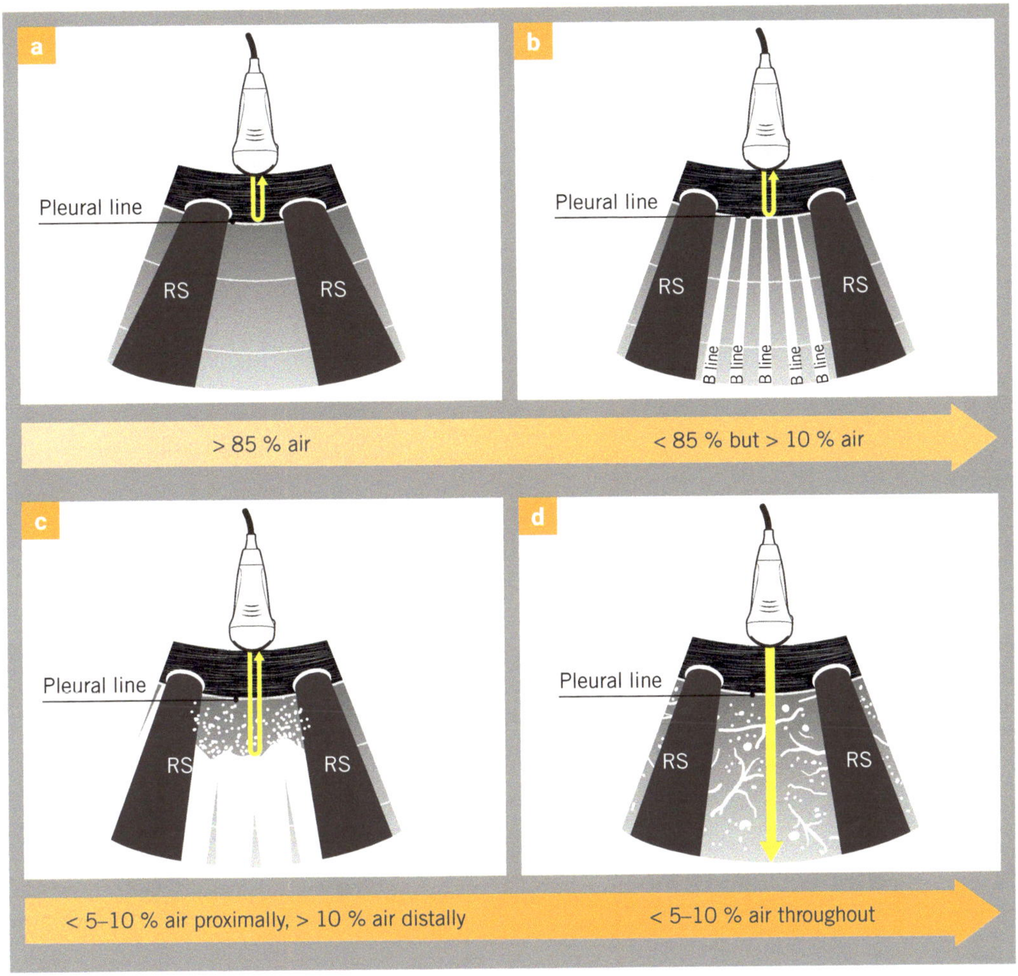

Figure 2. Schematic ultrasound images depicting different ratios of aerated to non-aerated lung, and the interaction of the ultrasound beam with the lung surface and underlying lung tissues at the lung surface. When the lung contains > 85 % air below the lung surface (normal aerated lung), the ultrasound beam is reflected from the soft tissue air interface (yellow curved arrow) that is normally present at the pleural line. This makes the lung tissue below the pleural line invisible to ultrasound, although artifacts such as A lines (depicted) may be visible (shown) (a). An example of lung that contains < 85 % but > 10 % air just below the lung surface. The ultrasound beam is reflected from the pleural line (yellow curved arrow) and the lung is not sonographically visible; however, artifact that represents underlying lung pathology is visible at the lung surface (five B lines in this example) (b). A region of lung that contains < 5–10 % air below the lung surface is depicted. When this situation is encountered the lung becomes sonographically visible as lung consolidation. Ultrasound beams will traverse consolidated lung tissue until they encounter a region of lung below the area of consolidation which contains more than 10 % air. This creates a new soft tissue-to-air interface that reflects the ultrasound beam (yellow curved arrow) back to the transducer, preventing lung below the distal border of consolidation from being sonographically visible (c). In this example the ultrasound beam (straight yellow arrow) does not encounter a region of aerated lung below the consolidation with > 10 % air, which allows the beams to continue to pass through the consolidated lung tissue. Ultrasound beams will continue to travel through regions of lung consolidation until they either encounter more aerated lung (> 10 % air) or they reach the distal surface of the lung (d).

Lung consolidation is not an artifact and is a true sonographic visualization of abnormal lung tissue.

When the ratio of aerated to non-aerated lung tissue directly below the visceral pleura falls below 5–10 %, the acoustic impedance between the thoracic wall and lung is decreased and there is a shift from the pleura, acting as a mirror and reflecting the ultrasound beam, to the ultrasound beam traversing the pleura and travelling through the underlying lung tissues[6]. Once the normal soft tissue-to-air interface at the pleural line is lost, ultrasound beams will continue to travel through consolidated lung tissue until one of two situations is encountered:

- The ultrasound beam encounters a section of lung below the consolidation that contains a ratio of more than 5–10 % aerated to non-aerated tissue (Figs. 2c and 3; video 7.1).
- The ultrasound beam traverses the entire width of the lung lobe (Figs. 2d and 4; video 7.2).

When the lung becomes sonographically visible it is referred to as lung consolidation and is often referred to as being "tissue-like" or "hepatized" as it resembles the tissue echogenicity of liver[7].

With partial lung ultrasound consolidation, ring down artifact will often be seen extending distally from the site the ultrasound beam encounters the distal border of the consolidated tissue (Fig. 3; video 7.3). This artifact extends to the far field of the ultrasound image and moves in sync with the consolidated lung tissue. The specific cause and significance of this ring down artifact has not been investigated; depending on the associated PLUS findings and lung pathology present it may represent similar pathology to increased B lines, or it may arise from a mechanism independent of B line formation.

QR
Video 7.1.
Shred sign, partial lung consolidation.

QR
Video 7.2.
Full translobar hepatization.

QR
Video 7.3.
Partial lung consolidation with distal border ring down artifact.

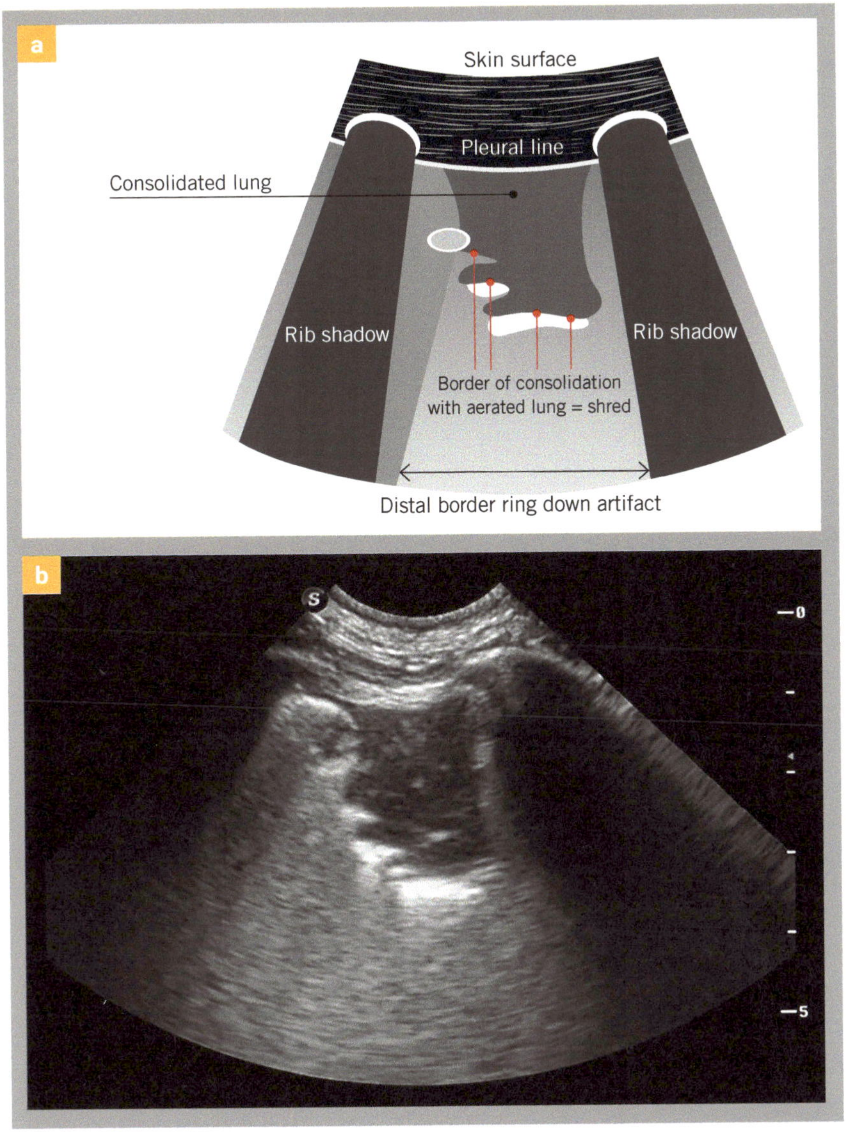

Figure 3. Schematic (a) and still ultrasound (b) images of ring down artifact arising from the distal border of partial lung consolidation. With all forms of non-translobar lung consolidation the acoustic window created by lung pathology encounters a higher percentage of air-filled lung deep to the pathology which reflects the ultrasound beam. At the site where the ultrasound beam is reflected, ring down artifact (lighter shaded area) can often be seen. Although this ring down artifact may move in sync with the respiratory cycle, unlike true B lines, it does not arise from the lung surface; it arises from the deep border of lung consolidation. This ring down artifact has not been well studied and further research is needed to determine its significance. Red lines delineate the border between consolidated lung and deeper more air-filled lung. The absence of A lines and presence of ring down artifact is seen deep to the consolidated tissue.

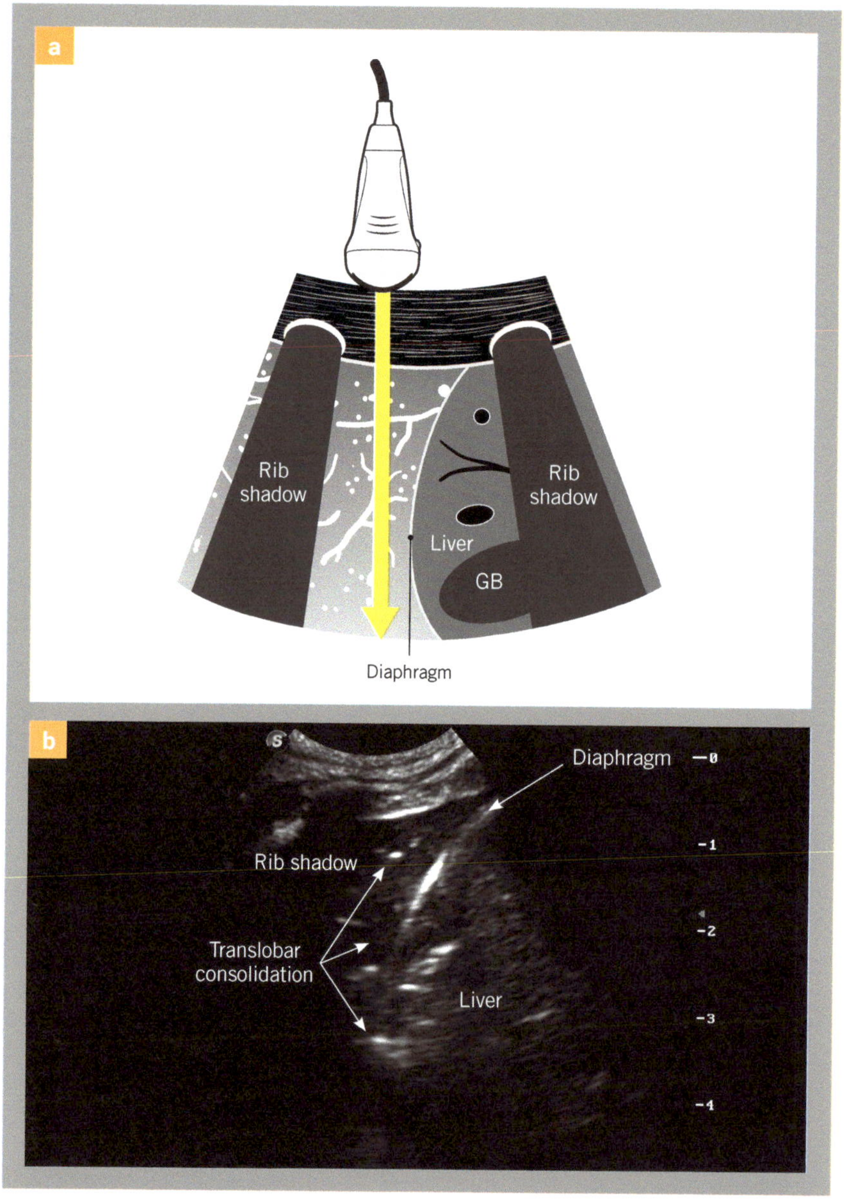

Figure 4. Schematic (a) and still ultrasound (b) image of translobar lung consolidation. The soft tissue-to-aerated lung interface at the pleural line is lost and consolidated lung is visible throughout the ultrasound image. The ultrasound beam (yellow arrow) will continue to travel through consolidated lung tissue as there is no soft tissue-to-air interface encountered below the consolidated lung region to reflect the beam back to the ultrasound transducer. Therefore, consolidation will be visible between the proximal and distal lung surfaces, extending to the far field of the ultrasound image as shown. A lines are not visible within consolidated regions of the lung. With translobar consolidation both the proximal and distal borders of the lung lobe are visible; in this image the proximal lung border is located at the thoracic wall and the distal border is along the diaphragm. GB; gallbladder.

Unlike B lines, the identification of lung consolidation, regardless of size, is always significant. However, like B lines, lung consolidation is non-specific; it is a common end pathway resulting from an increase in the proportion of non-aerated lung tissue. As stated previously (see Chapter 6), an increase in non-aerated lung tissue can be absolute or relative:

- **Absolute increases** are often the result of increased extravascular lung water (EVLW) or less commonly increased cell numbers (e.g. neoplasia, inflammatory cells, etc) or tissue (e.g. fibrous tissue).
- **Relative increases** are due to underinflation or collapse of alveoli (Fig. 1).

The most common causes of lung ultrasound consolidations include inflammatory conditions associated with increased EVLW, such as pulmonary contusions, acute respiratory distress syndrome (ARDS), and bronchopneumonia[2]. Other reported causes of lung ultrasound consolidation that may or may not be associated with increased EVLW include dynamic airway collapse, atelectasis, neoplasia, pulmonary thromboembolism and granulomatous diseases[2]. Pulmonary edema secondary to fluid overload and left sided congestive heart failure does not appear to be a common cause of lung ultrasound consolidation, although research including more severe cases of congestive heart failure in small animals is lacking. While ultrasound can diagnose consolidations (image finding), only clinicians can determine the cause (clinical diagnosis) by combining ultrasound findings with available clinical information, thereby directing further interventions and therapy.

Key concepts

- Applying PLUS allows identification of lung consolidation with minimal risk to patient safety.
- Lung consolidations can be identified over any lung region; perform a complete PLUS evaluation to decrease the likelihood of missing focal lesions.
- Lung consolidation occurs when air that usually fills the alveoli and small airways is lost or replaced by fluid, cells or tissue; it becomes sonographically visible when lung tissue directly below the lung surface contains less than 5–10 % air.
- Lung consolidation is a common end pathway of many disease processes.
- Different causes of lung consolidation can look similar on ultrasound; signalment, history, clinical examination and complementary diagnostics, as well as lesion distribution help determine the underlying cause.
- Assessing the different characteristics of lung consolidation may allow the differential diagnosis to be further refined.

CRITERIA TO DIAGNOSE LUNG CONSOLIDATION

The identification of hypoechoic lung parenchyma extending from the lung surface towards the far field of the ultrasound image indicates peripheral lung consolidation.

Criteria to rule out lung consolidation

Definitively ruling out lung consolidation with ultrasound alone is not possible for several reasons:

- Lung consolidations can be focal. It is not possible to scan the entire lung surface due to limitations imposed by the anatomic structure of the thorax (only about 2/3 of the lung surface and about 1/16th of the total lung can be sonographically visualized)[8]. To minimize missing pathology, as much of the lung surface as possible should be scanned if focal consolidation is suspected. Performing a complete standardized PLUS exam is recommended (see Chapter 2).
- When more diffuse consolidation is suspected the experienced clinician may be more selective regarding which lung regions to initially scan, depending on the concurrent history and clinical findings. For example, with increased crackles auscultated over the right cranial ventral thorax in a dog presenting with respiratory distress and a history of vomiting the clinician may start by scanning the cranial ventral lung regions for lung consolidation secondary to aspiration pneumonia before completing the PLUS and other POCUS examinations.
- Given lung ultrasound is a surface imaging technique, it is not possible to rule out lung consolidation at a specific transducer location if the lung consolidation fails to reach the lung surface at that site (Fig. 5). However, according to human research, > 90 % of inflammatory causes of lung consolidation, which are the most common forms, reach the lung surface[7]. This is also likely true in small animal patients.

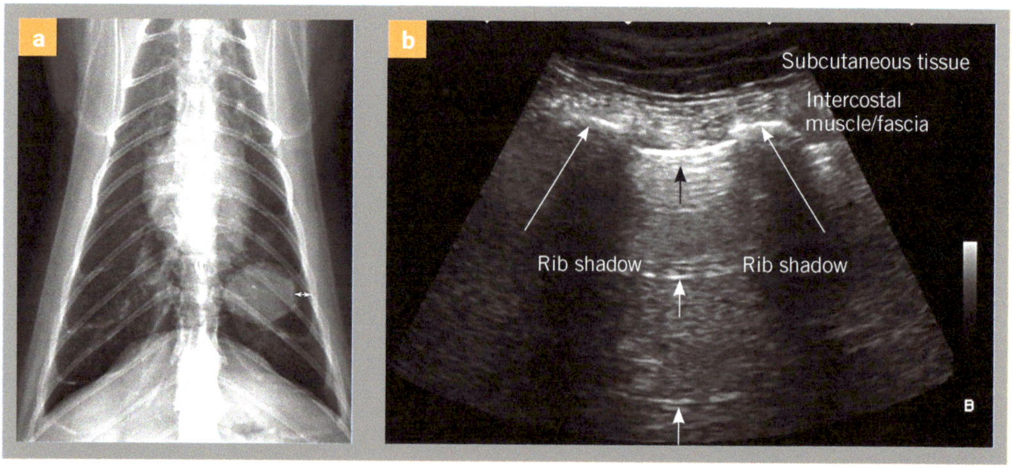

Figure 5. Dorsoventral thoracic radiograph (lateral radiograph not shown) (a) and still ultrasound image from a cat diagnosed with a lung mass that is separated from the lateral lung surface by air-filled lung (white double headed arrow) (b). Ultrasound will fail to detect the mass in this patient because a soft tissue-to-air interface is present lateral to the mass resulting in the "bat sign" and normal dry lung air artifact.

Criteria to rule in lung consolidation

The sonographic confirmation of lung consolidation is based on the following three criteria[7]:

- A superficial border is present.
- A hypoechoic tissue-like echogenicity is present.
- A deep boundary is present.

A superficial border is present

The lung surface forms the superficial border of consolidation.

All sonographically visible lung consolidation must arise from the lung surface:

- Consolidations will arise from the pleural line when the lung is in contact with the thoracic wall.
- Consolidations will arise from the lung surface, distal to the pleural line and separated from the thoracic wall if pleural fluid or a pleural mass is present within the pleural space (Fig. 6; video 7.4).
- If air separates the lung surface from the thoracic wall (e.g. pneumothorax), the lung will not be visible and it is therefore not possible to assess if lung consolidation is present or absent at that transducer location.

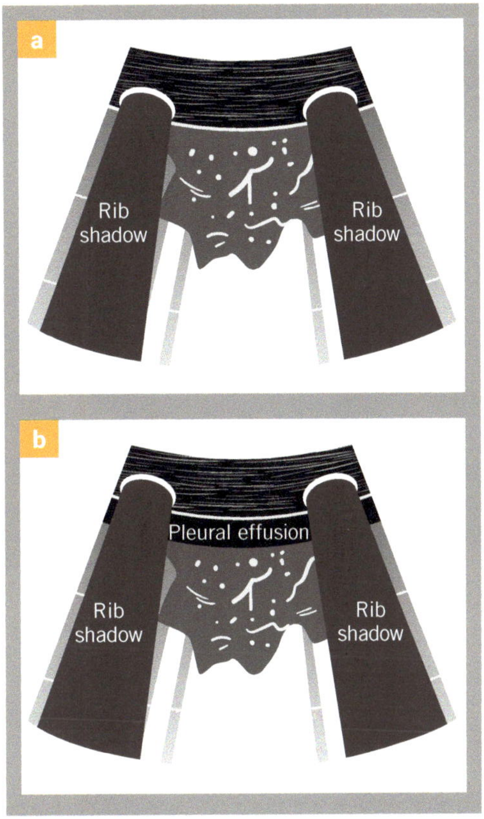

Figure 6. Schematic ultrasound images of visible lung consolidations arising from the lung surface. Consolidations will arise from the pleural line when the lung is in contact with the thoracic wall. Consolidations will arise from the lung surface, separated from the thoracic wall, if pleural fluid (or a pleural mass) is present within the pleural space (b). Consolidation should be interpreted with caution when separated from the thoracic wall as passive atelectasis can create consolidation that is difficult to differentiate from intrapulmonary lung pathology (see atelectasis below). Serial evaluation should be performed, particularly after resolution of pleural space pathology that might be causing passive atelectasis.

QR
Video 7.4.
Consolidated lung deep to fluid.

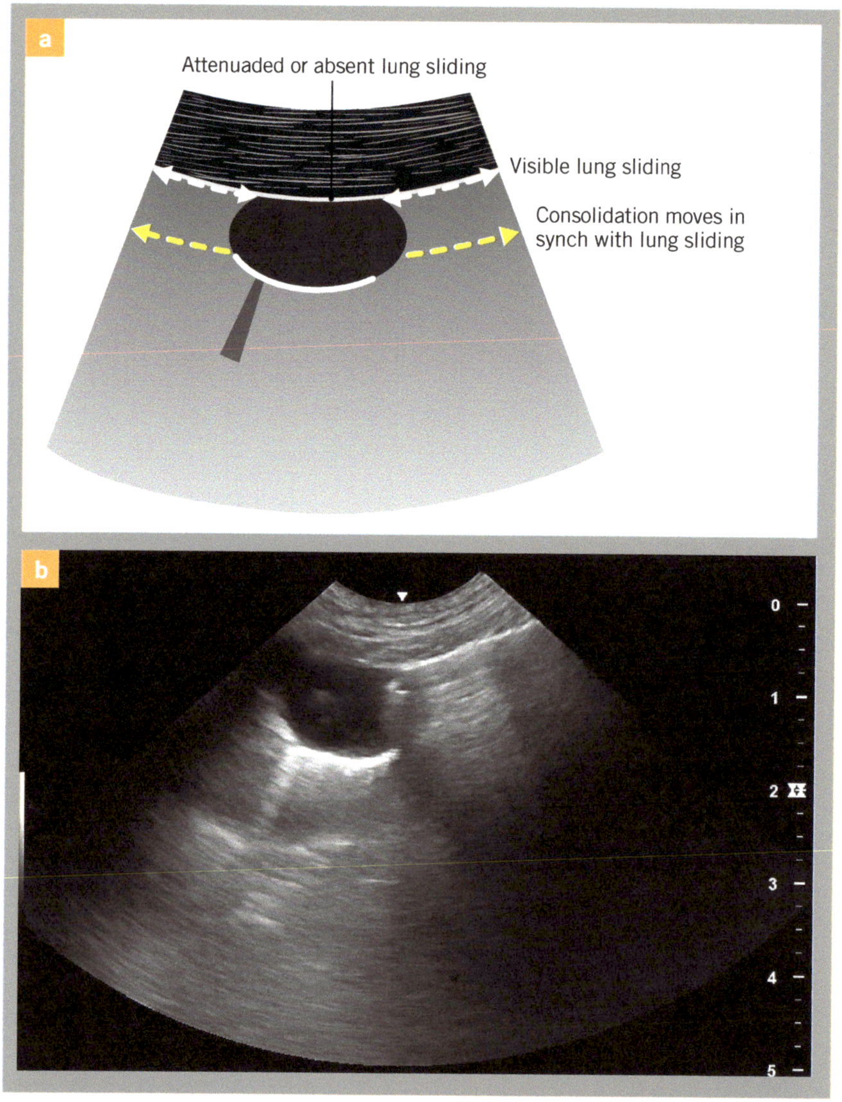

Figure 7. Schematic and still ultrasound images of a partial lung consolidation, in this case a nodule. White dotted arrows indicate the presence of visible lung sliding to either side of the nodule. The parietal pleura may be visible where lung consolidation contacts the thoracic wall; however, lung sliding will be attenuated to absent (depicted in the schematic by the absence of dotted lines). Despite the absence of visible lung sliding between the nodule and thoracic wall, the area of consolidation will still move in sync with the visible lung sliding to either side of the nodule (yellow dotted arrows indicate movement of the nodule in synch with lung sliding).

It can sometimes be difficult to differentiate mirror/reverberation artifact below the pleural line from lung consolidation. However, there are a few tricks that can help differentiate the two:

- Smaller lung ultrasound consolidations, because they are contained within the lung and arise from the lung surface, will move in sync with the respiratory cycle if there is sufficient lung expansion to create lung sliding (Fig. 7; video 7.5).
- In contrast, mirror image/reverberation artifact will not move in sync with lung sliding; mirror image/reverberation artifact may move slightly in sync with the intercostal muscle and subcutaneous tissues they mirror, but it will be independent of lung sliding (Fig. 8; video 7.6).

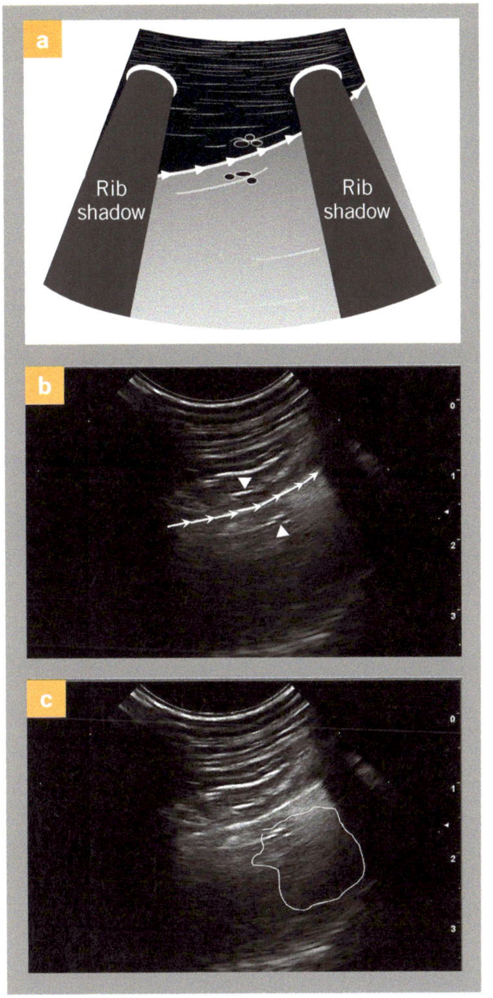

Figure 8. Schematic and still ultrasound images of mirror/reverberation artifact. Schematic image demonstrating how structures located above the pleural line can be mirrored below the pleural line giving the false impression of consolidated lung tissue (a). By observing lung sliding along the pleural line (white arrows), it is apparent that the mirrored artifacts do not move in synch with lung sliding. The mirrored artifact also fails to reach the lung surface and there is no attenuation of the pleural line above the area of mirrored artifact. Labelled still image of the schematic (b). An area is outlined on the ultrasound still image that might be mistaken as having a "tissue-like" appearance and therefore confused for consolidation (c); however, the region does not reach the lung surface and does not move in sync with lung sliding.

QR
Video 7.5.
Consolidation moving with the lung surface.

QR
Video 7.6.
Mirror image not moving with the lung surface.

Lung sliding may be diminished or absent at the superficial border of consolidation that is in contact with the thoracic wall.

- The pleural line is often attenuated or obliterated over areas of partial lung consolidation; therefore, lung sliding is often not visible between the thoracic wall and partial lung consolidations. Where lung sliding is visible along the pleural line, consolidation will appear to move in sync with lung sliding (Fig. 7; video 7.7).
- In cases of complete lung lobe consolidation there is often no visible lung expansion during the respiratory cycle and therefore an absence of lung sliding (Fig. 9; video 7.8)[3].

QR
Video 7.7.
Attenuated pleural line with consolidation.

A hypoechoic "tissue-like" echogenicity is present

A number of tissue-like patterns can occur which vary depending on the presence or absence of hyperechoic air bronchograms or anechoic fluid bronchograms (see below).

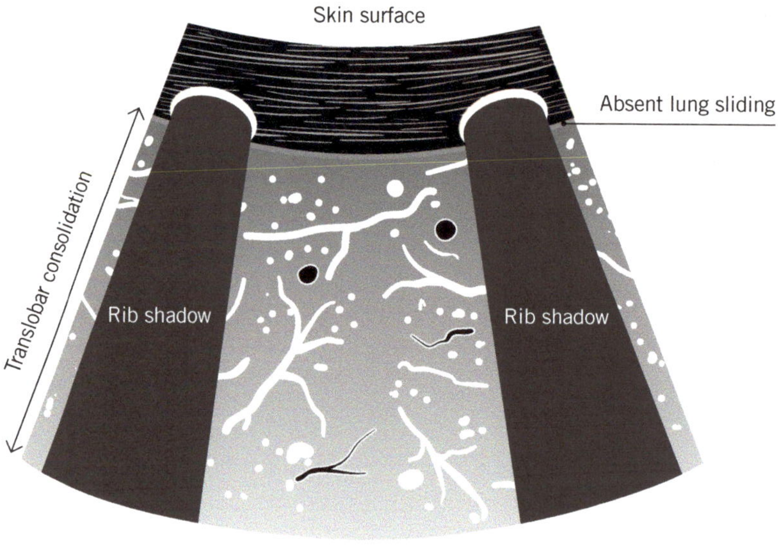

Figure 9. Schematic ultrasound image of translobar lung consolidation. When translobar consolidation is present and extensive (e.g. most of the lung lobe is affected), there may be insufficient inflation and deflation of the lung to create visible lung sliding. Air movement may be visible within the lung (dynamic air bronchograms, see below). However movement of the lung along the thoracic wall may be absent.

A deep boundary is present

- If the tissue-like pattern does not traverse the entire width of the lung lobe it is considered partial (non-translobar), and the deep boundary is defined by the transition from the consolidated lung to aerated lung below the consolidated region (Fig. 3; video 7.1)[7].
- If the tissue-like pattern traverses the entire width of the lung lobe at that transducer location it is termed translobar, and the deep boundary is defined by the opposite lung surface (Fig. 4; video 7.2)[7].
- With partial consolidations the aerated lung tissue situated below the consolidation will not be visible (Fig. 3), while the width of the entire lung lobe is visible with translobar consolidations, at the transducer location (Fig. 4).

It is important to note that within a lung or lung lobe, consolidation may occur focally or diffusely. As such partial and translobar lung consolidation, as well as normal lung and increased B lines, or any combination thereof, may be present within the same lung lobe or even the same ultrasound window (Fig. 10; video 7.9).

QR
Video 7.8.
Absent lung sliding and pleura line attenuation with consolidation.

QR
Video 7.9.
Combined partial and translobar consolidation in the same window.

Criteria to rule in or out lung consolidations

Rule in findings	Rule out findings
A superficial border is present.	Lung sliding with A lines and/or ≤ 3 B lines. However: - Cannot fully rule out deeper consolidations. - Cannot scan the entire lung due to anatomical challenges.
A hypoechoic tissue-like echogenicity is present.	
A deep boundary is present.	

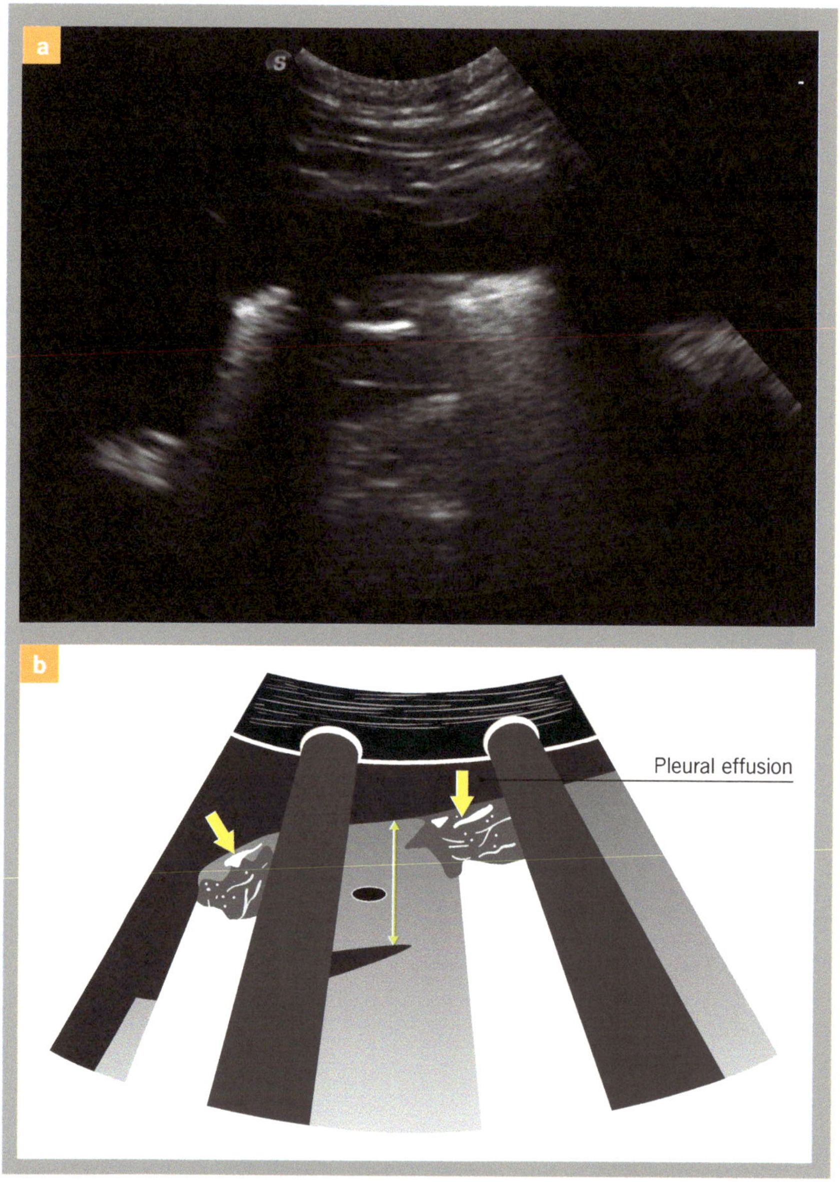

Figure 10. Still and schematic ultrasound images of partial and translobar consolidation within the same lung lobe and ultrasound window. In this example, the consolidation is due to compressive atelectasis. The yellow double-headed arrow represents a region of translobar consolidation while the yellow arrowheads represent partial consolidation (shred signs in this case). Note that the tissues are visible through the far field below the translobar lung consolidation as there is no aerated lung encountered to reflect the ultrasound beam. The regions below the right and left sided partial consolidations are obscured by ring down artifact that arises from the consolidation to aerated lung border, preventing the far field from being interpreted. Also note there is a single round fluid bronchogram visible within the middle region of the translobar consolidation.

CRITERIA TO CHARACTERIZE LUNG CONSOLIDATIONS

There are five key questions that should be considered to further characterize the consolidation. Answering these binary/closed questions at each PLUS sonographic window helps narrow the differential list for causes of lung consolidation. In addition, mapping the patterns visible within and between different PLUS regions creates a PLUS profile for the patient, which also helps determine the underlying cause (see ultrasound lung profiles below).

Is the consolidation partial (non-translobar) or translobar?

As mentioned, there are two general classifications used to describe the depth of lung consolidation at a specific transducer location:

- Partial (or non-translobar) consolidation occurs when the ultrasound beam encounters a new soft tissue-to-air interface within a lung lobe deep to the consolidation (where aerated lung reflects the ultrasound beam back to the transducer) (Fig. 3)[7].
- Translobar consolidation occurs when the ultrasound beam traverses the entire width of the lung lobe from the superficial surface to the distal surface without encountering significantly aerated lung tissue (aerated to non-aerated ratio is ≤ 5–10 % across the width of the lung lobe) (Fig. 4)[7].

Translobar consolidation represent a more severe form of lung consolidation relative to partial consolidation as there is a lack of aerated lung throughout the width of the lung lobe at the transducer location; however, their differential diagnoses are similar.

Partial consolidations: is it a shred, nodule or wedge sign?

When partial (non-translobar) consolidations are present, they can be further classified into three subcategories depending on their shape[1,9-11], characteristics of the interface between partial consolidation and underlying aerated lung, and the characteristics within the area of consolidation. These three classifications (Fig. 11) are:

- Shred signs (video 7.1).
- Nodule signs (video 7.10).
- Wedge signs (video 7.11).

The three classifications of partial consolidation are not mutually exclusive, and any combination can be found in a patient, which emphasizes the need to scan multiple regions and to consider the entire PLUS profile in conjunction with history and other clinical findings.

Pleural thickening is often considered an early form of consolidation (Fig. 11d).

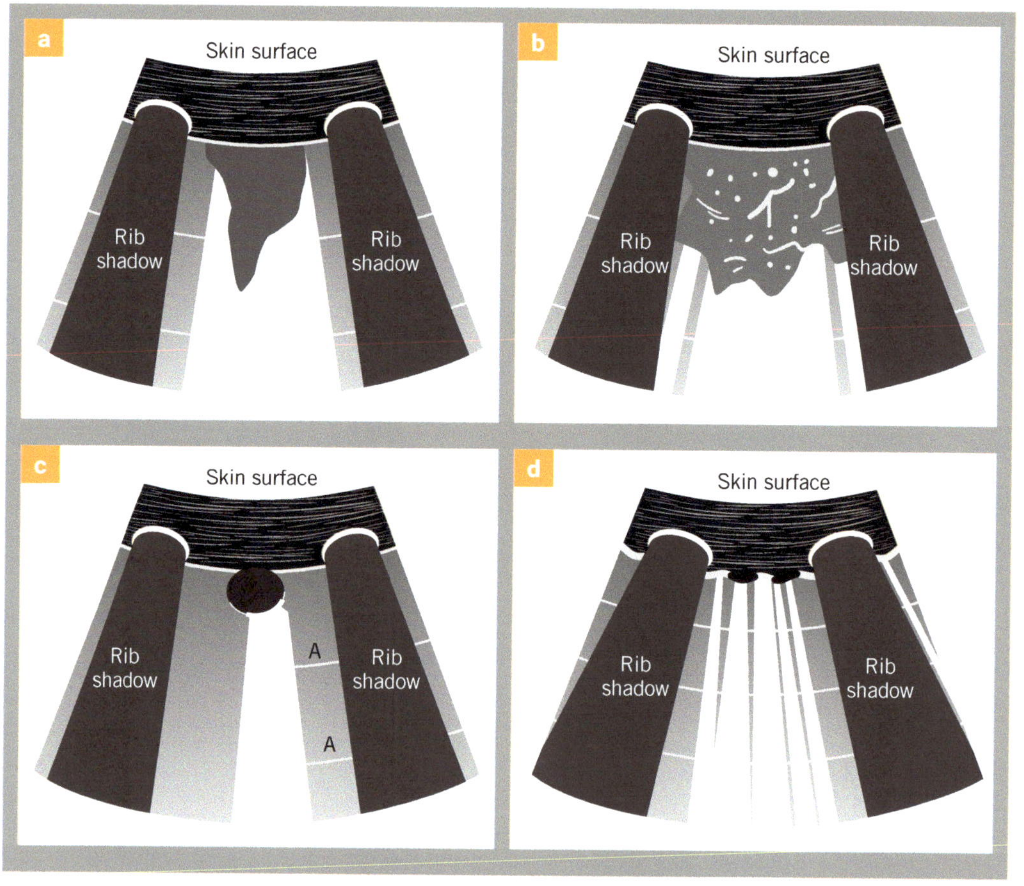

Figure 11. Schematic ultrasound images of subpleural consolidation and thickening seen with different underlying pathologies. A classic wedge or triangular shaped consolidation that lacks air bronchograms and has a relatively smooth hyperechoic and well-demarcated border is typical of pulmonary embolism, particularly if these lesions are located at 2–3 lung sites with appropriate supporting history and clinical findings (a). The shred sign can vary in size and has a rough broken and often poorly defined distal border. Shred signs often contain air and/or fluid bronchograms (see below) (b). The classic nodule sign has a well-defined smooth hyperechoic semicircular to oval border and is often found with neoplasia, fungal and other nodular diseases, and lung surface abscesses (c). Pleural thickening is a fairly nonspecific finding that appears as thickening of the pleural line, often having a "moth eaten" appearance and is considered by some to be an early sign of lung consolidation (d). A; A line.

QR
Video 7.10.
Nodule sign.

QR
Video 7.11.
"Wedge sign".

The "shred sign" (also referred to as the fractal sign)

A "shred sign" is a partial consolidation that appears as if "chunks" have been taken out of the lung creating echo poor areas. With this type of partial consolidation, the junction from consolidated lung to aerated lung is very irregular, hyperechoic, serrated and blurred, creating a "shred" like appearance similar to a "torn" or shredded piece of paper (Figs. 11c and 12a)[7-11]. Although research is lacking in veterinary medicine, the "shred sign" is most likely associated with pneumonia, but can also occur as a result of hemorrhage (e.g. traumatic pulmonary contusions) and other inflammatory causes of increased EVLW, or less often by neoplastic or thromboembolic disease.

Assessing the characteristics of the tissue consolidation of a "shred sign" may help differentiate the "shred sign" from other causes of partial lung consolidation.

The consolidated lung tissue comprising a "shred sign" often contains punctate to linear hyperechoic air bronchograms or hypoechoic fluid bronchograms, which tend to be absent within "nodule" and "wedge signs" (see bronchograms below).

Assessing adjacent regions of lung surrounding a "shred sign" as well as the pleural space helps create the PLUS profile for the patient, and is helpful in determining the underlying cause (Figs. 13–15; table 1; video 7.12).

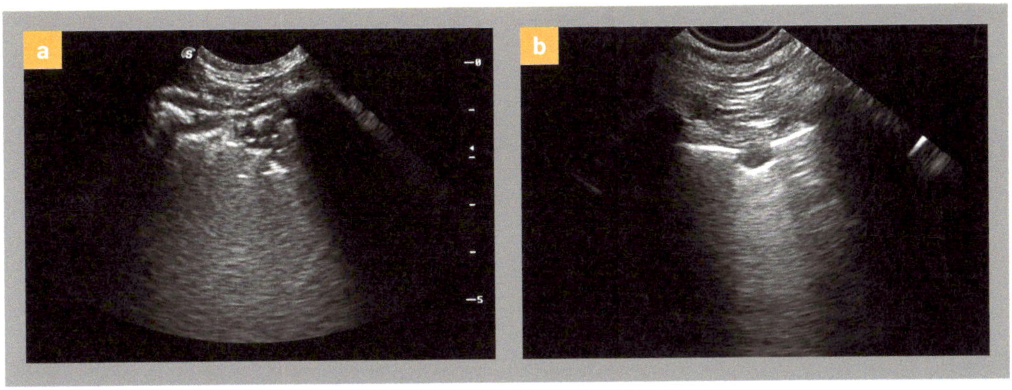

Figure 12. Still ultrasound images of a shred sign (a) that shows a "broken" blurred distal border and punctate hyperechoic air bronchograms within the partially consolidated lung tissue compared to a "nodule sign" (b) which classically shows a more defined distal smooth border and the absence of air bronchograms within the consolidated lung tissue.

QR

Video 7.12.
PLUS profile
aspiration pneumonia
in a Great Dane.

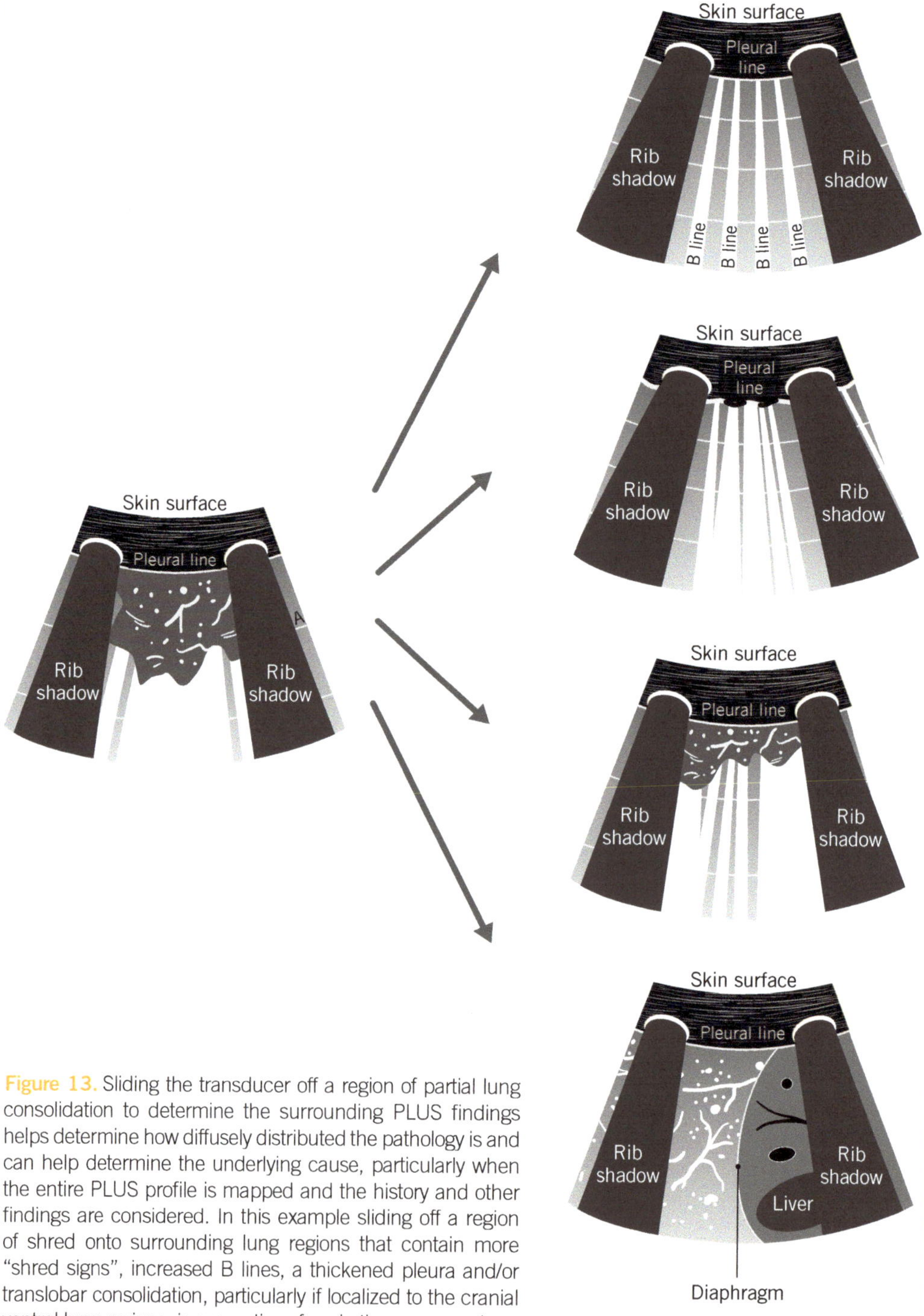

Figure 13. Sliding the transducer off a region of partial lung consolidation to determine the surrounding PLUS findings helps determine how diffusely distributed the pathology is and can help determine the underlying cause, particularly when the entire PLUS profile is mapped and the history and other findings are considered. In this example sliding off a region of shred onto surrounding lung regions that contain more "shred signs", increased B lines, a thickened pleura and/or translobar consolidation, particularly if localized to the cranial ventral lung regions, is suggestive of aspiration pneumonia.

- If the transducer is slid off a region of lung containing a "shred sign" onto adjacent regions where increased B lines, and a thickened irregular pleura, consolidation or a combination of these are seen, pneumonia, hemorrhage and ARDS should be considered (Fig. 13). Further history and the entire PLUS profile with the characterization and distribution of lesions should be determined.
- In contrast, regions adjacent to an isolated partial lung consolidation that display only lung sliding with A lines (normal pleura & no B lines) makes the partial consolidation unlikely to be a "shred sign"; nodular and thromboembolic diseases should be considered (Fig. 14). However, considerable overlap exists, emphasizing the importance of history and other clinical findings.

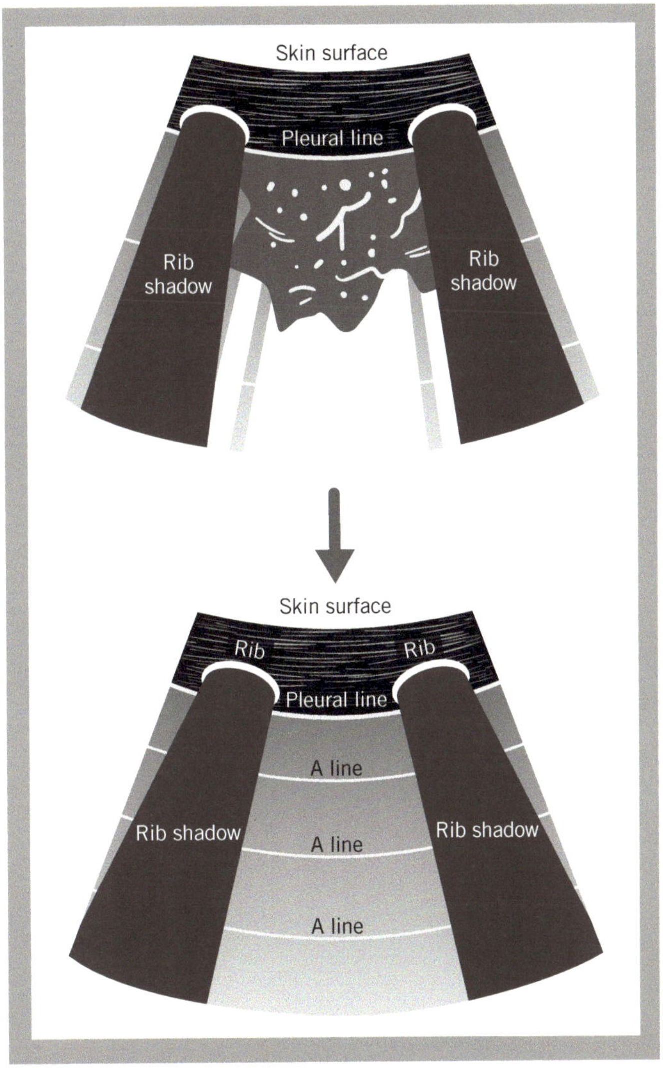

Figure 14. Sliding the transducer off a region of partial lung consolidation onto surrounding lung regions helps determine how diffusely distributed the pathology is and can help determine the underlying cause, particularly when the entire PLUS profile is mapped and the history and other findings are considered. In this example sliding off a region of partial consolidation onto surrounding lung regions that contain only lung sliding and A lines in the absence of other abnormal PLUS findings would be consistent with a nodule or pulmonary thromboembolism, and less likely pneumonia or ARDS, which tend to be diffuse and have mixed PLUS profiles.

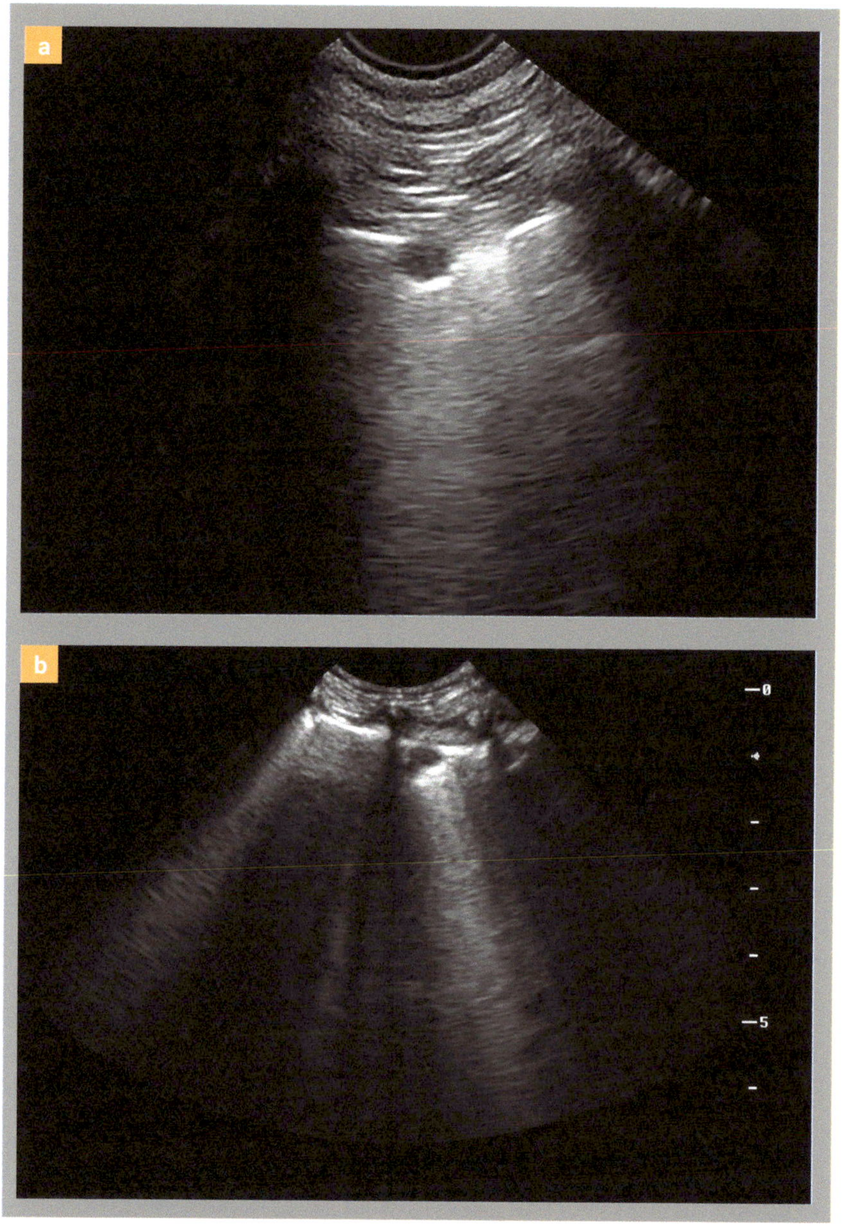

Figure 15. Two very similar partial lung consolidations from two different patients. Nodule secondary to metastatic neoplasia (a). Note the regions of lung cranial and caudal to the nodule are dry. The region to the right of the nodule contains a few A lines and there are no B lines visible in the image, although a ring down artifact originates from the distal border of the nodule. The lungs were considered dry throughout all regions in this patient. Image from a dog with aspiration pneumonia (b). Note the regions cranial and caudal to the partially consolidated lung contain B lines. There is also a ring down artifact originating from the distal border of the partial consolidation. The partial consolidation to the right is an "atypical" shred sign as it has a fairly delineated distal border. In isolation, it would be easy to confuse the two consolidations; however, consideration of all PLUS ultrasound findings within the ultrasound window as well as multiple PLUS regions helps create a bigger picture to narrow down the differential diagnosis.

The "nodule sign"

A "nodule sign" is a type of partial consolidation defined by the presence of a smooth hypoechoic or moderately echogenic region that is well delineated, and often has a semicircular, oval, to circular deep boundary (Figs. 16 and 17; videos 7.10 and 7.13)[9-11]. Nodules often have a focal or multifocal distribution over the lung surface. Similar to the finding of nodules on radiographs the sonographic detection of nodules is suggestive of neoplasia, or less frequently of granulomatous disease, or even abscessation[9-11]. Ultrasound criteria alone are not sufficient to discriminate between primary tumor, metastasis, fungal disease and abscesses. However, careful assessment of the echogenic characteristics of a nodule can help differentiate it from other partial consolidations such as a shred sign: unlike shred signs nodules tend to be more homogenous in appearance, lacking air and fluid bronchograms (see below) which may be seen with shred and translobar signs. The adjacent tissue to either side of nodules should be sonographically assessed as it will often appear normal (lung sliding and no B lines or only A lines) in many cases (Fig. 15a), which is in contrast to most causes of shred signs (ARDS, hemorrhage, pneumonia, etc.) which tend to be associated with increased B lines (Fig. 15b)[11,12]. If the underlying neoplasia is associated with increased EVLW (e.g. hemangiosarcoma), then increased B lines will likely be present.

QR

Video 7.13.
Different nodule – fungal.

- Note: "Nodule signs" are only one form of consolidation seen with neoplasia and it is possible to see shred and translobar consolidation with neoplastic processes, depending on the underlying cause of neoplasia. Although less common, neoplastic consolidations may occasionally contain air bronchograms, which emphasizes interpreting finding in light of history and all PLUS findings.

The "wedge sign"

A "wedge sign" (Fig. 18; video 7.11) is suggestive of pulmonary thromboembolism (PTE), with 85 % of sonographically identified pulmonary thromboembolic consolidations in humans having a wedge shape[13,14]. However, some patients will have rounded or polygonal shaped subpleural consolidations, which can be confused for "shred signs" and "nodule signs"[13,14]. Wedge shaped lesions are also observed with pathologies other than PTE. Therefore, the "wedge sign" is neither sensitive nor specific, and should be interpreted with caution[13,14]. The outer borders of the wedge are clearly delineated (in contrast to "shred signs" which are poorly defined), yet irregular in shape.

Several additional sonographic and clinical criteria are required to diagnose PTE induced consolidations; the diagnosis should not be made based on the finding of sonographic "wedge sign" alone.

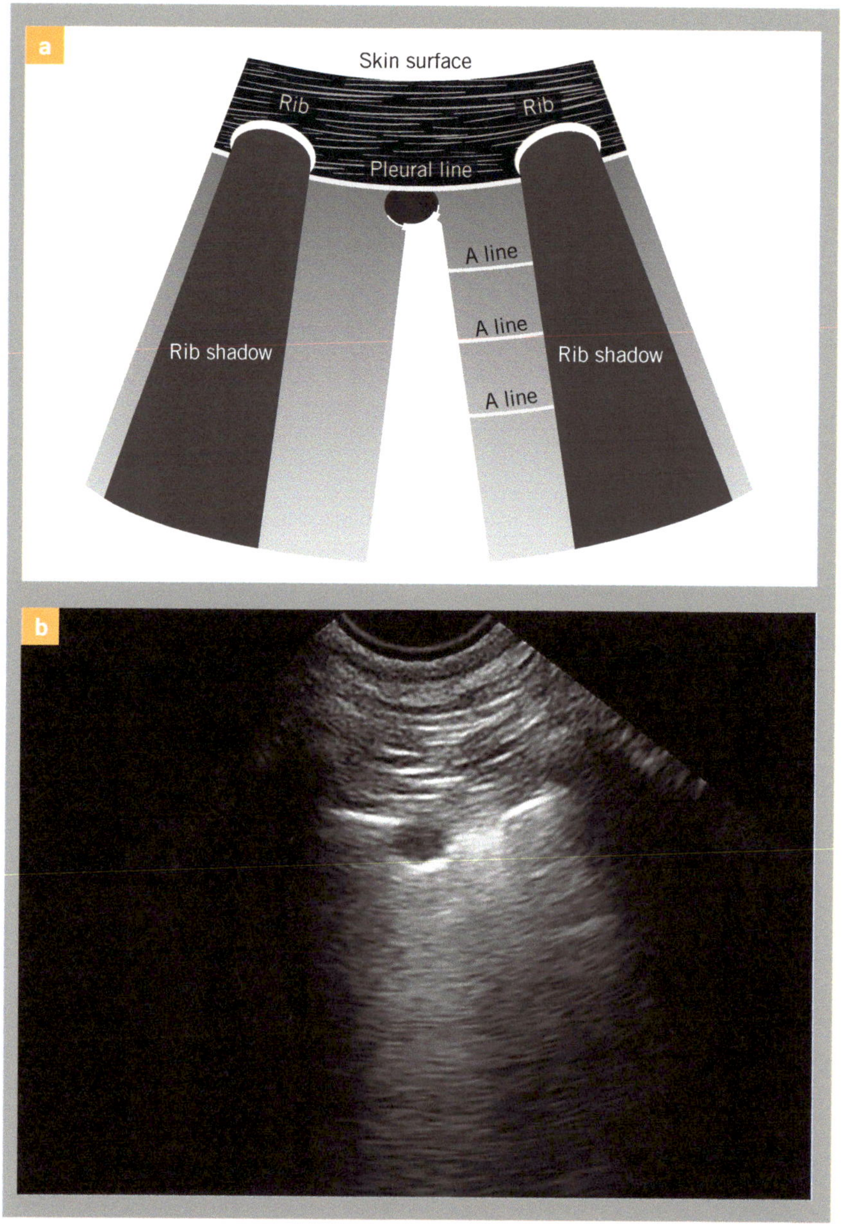

Figure 16. Schematic (a) and ultrasound still (b) image from an 8-year-old Golden Retriever that presented for a 1-week history of decreased activity and appetite. On ultrasound multiple round hypoechoic, well-delineated lesions were identified over various regions, consistent with a nodule sign. Note the absence of air bronchograms, homogenous nature of the consolidation and the well demarcated smooth borders, as well as ring down artifact arising from the distal wall and extending though the far field of the image. Unaffected lung is present to the right of the nodule extending to the rib shadow, which is indicated by the presence of A lines and lung sliding (not appreciated in a still image). A final diagnosis of lymphoma was based on biopsy of a nodule.

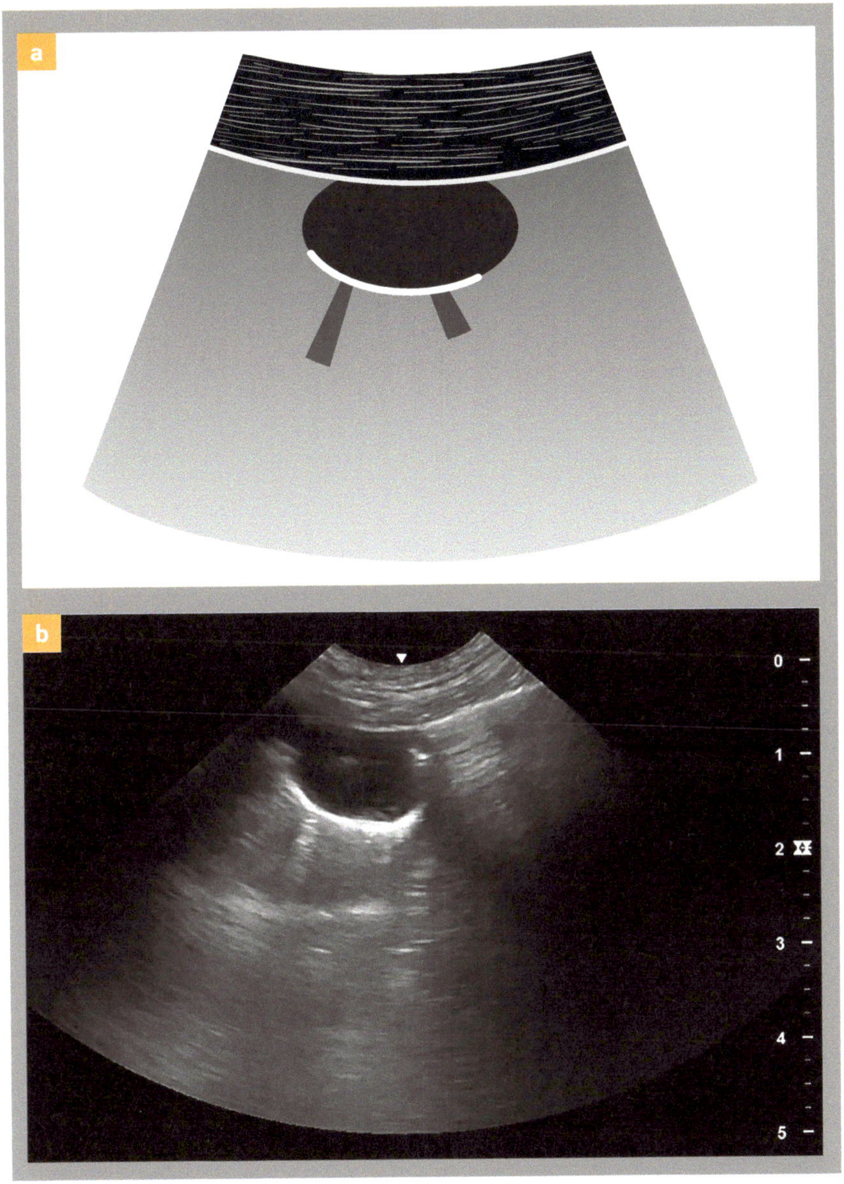

Figure 17. Schematic (a) and ultrasound still (b) images of 5-year-old mix breed canine that presented for cough and increased respiratory effort. A roughly 1 cm hypoechoic homogeneous round subpleural lesion with well demarcated smooth hyperechoic borders was identified. Note the absence of air bronchograms within the lesion. Rib shadows are not visible in the images as the transducer was orientated parallel to and angled under the rib to increase the lung surface evaluated during PLUS. Fine needle aspiration and cytology of the lesion confirmed blastomycosis. Similar to radiographs, it is not possible to distinguish neoplasia from fungal disease solely based on sonographic findings.

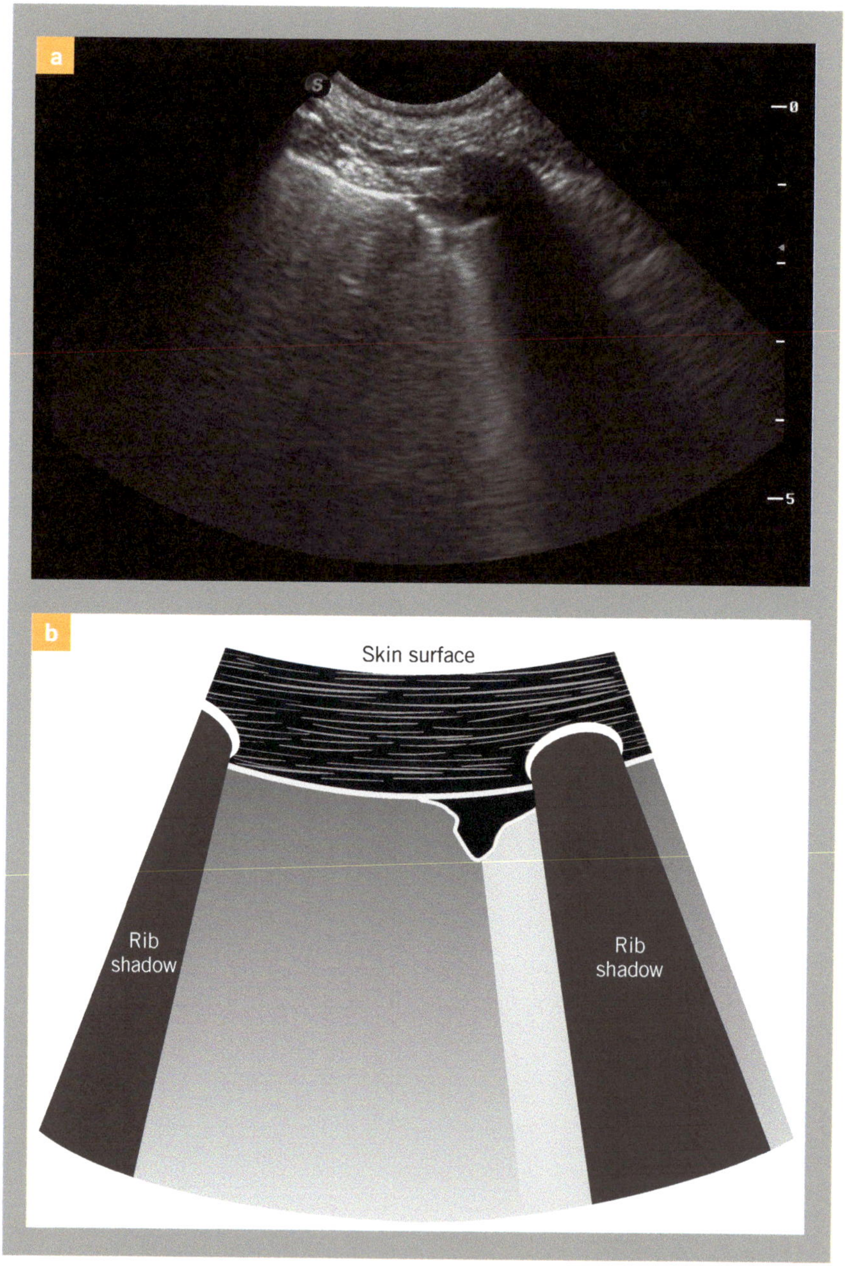

Figure 18. Still (a) and schematic (b) images of a "wedge sign". The detection of a wedge shaped partial lung consolidation on ultrasound should prompt consideration of pulmonary thromboembolism (PTE), although this is neither sensitive or specific and wedge shaped partial consolidations can be seen with other pathology other than PTE. The history, clinical findings and the entire PLUS profile should be considered when trying to decide if a wedge sign is due to PTE.

"Wedge sign" criteria in humans and corresponding comments for small animals

The following criteria are used in humans, but have not been investigated in companion animals[13,14]:

- In contrast to "shred signs", and similar to "nodule signs", "wedge signs" are homogeneous with an absence of air bronchograms, although a single central hyperechoic lesion may be present in a small number of cases.
- Gravity dependent lung regions are most affected:
  - It is unknown if gravity dependent regions are the most sensitive sites to identify sonographic PTE consolidations in veterinary patients. Given aspiration pneumonia is often identified at these sites, it is important to consider other lung ultrasound, history and clinical findings when interpreting gravity dependent lung consolidation.
  - The finding of wedge-shaped lesions in non-gravity dependent lung regions with other supporting history and clinical findings may be more supportive of PTE.
- The presence of wedge-shaped consolidations at more than two locations increases the specificity for pulmonary embolism.
- In contrast to "shred signs", surrounding inflammatory changes (e.g. B lines) are uncommon.
  - Due to species differences in disease mechanisms leading to prothrombotic states and species differences in pulmonary vasculature and anatomy, increased B lines may be more common in dogs and cats with sonographic PTE consolidations than in people.
- Sonographic pleural findings include localized fluid accumulation adjacent to the affected PTE consolidations, which eventually track to gravity dependent pleural sites.
  - The incidence of sonographically identified pleural effusion in veterinary patients with PTE is unknown.
- Vascular ultrasound assessment of consolidated lung lesions demonstrates an absence of blood flow using colour flow doppler.
  - It is difficult to have companion animals hold their breath and remain motionless; the application of colour flow doppler to assess lung lesions in companion animals is less practical.
- Detecting deep vein thrombosis on ultrasound increases the likelihood that "wedge signs" detected on lung ultrasound are due to PTE.
  - As sonographic identification of deep vein thrombosis is rare in veterinary patients with pulmonary thromboembolism, other clinicopathological findings and predisposing causes should be used to support the diagnosis.

Any small sonographic lung consolidation including "shred signs" and "nodule signs" can easily be confused for sonographic PTE consolidations. Moreover, the vasculature architecture of the lungs differs significantly between species. In the authors' experience, dogs suspected of pulmonary thromboembolism often present with increased B lines as opposed to lung consolidations.

In summary, PTE should be suspected in companion animals when isolated wedge-shaped consolidations, not associated with multiple "shred signs" or translobar consolidations, are identified in patients with a predisposing prothrombotic condition and other supporting history and clinical findings (e.g. hypercoagulable thromboelastographic tracing). In contrast, the finding of wedge shaped consolidations in conjunction with shred signs and translobar consolidations would be more suggestive of pneumonia. However, further research is required to determine the sonographic characteristics of PTE lesions, which lung regions are most sensitive for identification of PTE, and the overall accuracy of ultrasound for its detection.

Are air or fluid bronchograms present?

The appearance of lung ultrasound consolidation, particularly shred sign and translobar consolidations, can vary depending if the smaller airways still contain air (air bronchogram; video 7.14) or become flooded with fluid (fluid bronchogram; video 7.15) (Fig. 19)[9,10].

Air bronchograms appear as punctate or linear hyperechoic foci contained between the hyperechoic walls of bronchi, and are frequently seen in patients with various causes of shred and translobar consolidations (Fig. 20)[9,10].

Table 1. Partial lung lobe consolidations

Partial consolidation	Ultrasound appearance	Differential diagnosis
Shred	Appears as if "chunks" taken out of the lung creating echo poor areas; junction from consolidated lung to aerated lung very irregular, hyperechoic, serrated and blurred, creating a "shred" like appearance similar to a "torn" or shredded piece of paper.	Pneumonia Hemorrhage Inflammatory associated increases in extravascular lung water Thromboembolic disease Neoplasia
Nodule	Smooth hypoechoic or moderately echogenic region; well delineated, often has semicircular, oval, to circular deep boundary.	Fungal Primary or metastatic neoplasia Abscesses
Wedge	Wedge-shaped and often well delineated.	Pulmonary thromboembolism

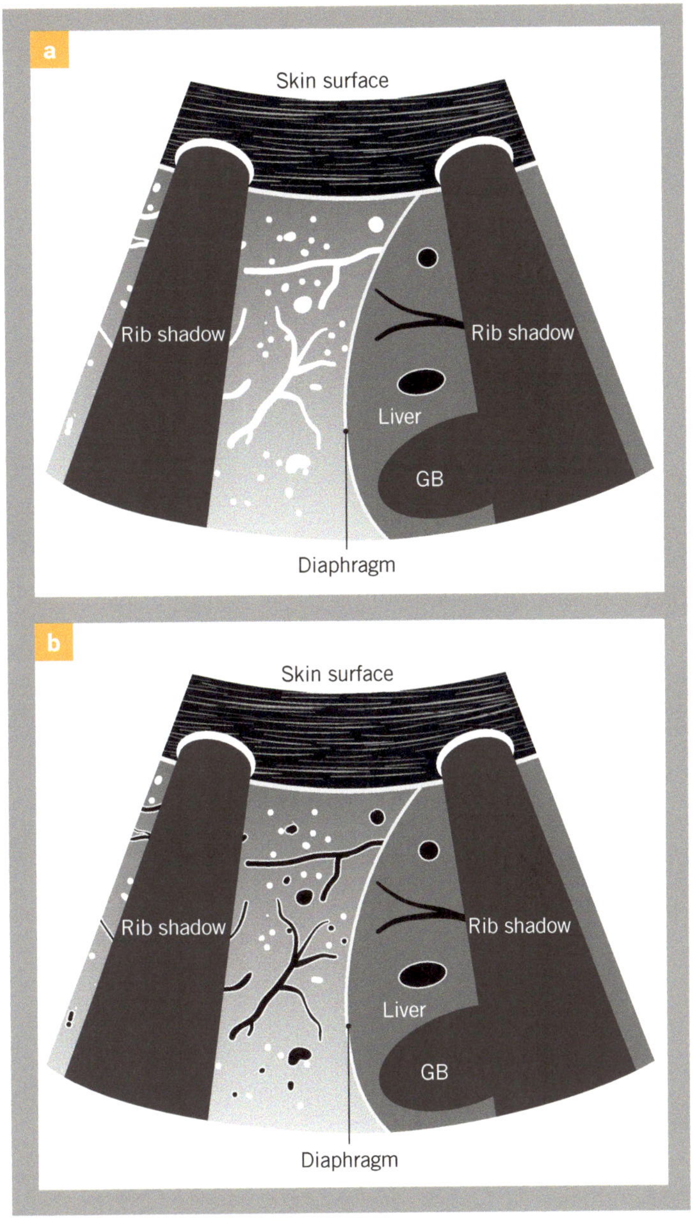

Figure 19. Schematic ultrasound images depicting the difference between air and fluid bronchograms. A translobar consolidation is shown with white hyperechoic punctate to linear structures representing air within bronchioles, referred to as air bronchograms (a). Air bronchograms are classified as static (no visible air movement within the air bronchogram) and dynamic (air visible moving within the air bronchogram during respiration). Fluid bronchograms appear as hypoechoic to anechoic punctate or linear structures and are sonographically visible when the airways become fluid filled (seen when air is replaced by fluid or inflammatory exudate) (b). It is possible to find both fluid and air bronchograms within the same consolidated region of lung or in different regions of a lung lobe. They can be detected in both shred and translobar consolidations, but tend to be absent with nodule and wedge signs. GB; gallbladder.

QR
Video 7.14.
Air bronchogram.

QR
Video 7.15.
Fluid bronchogram.

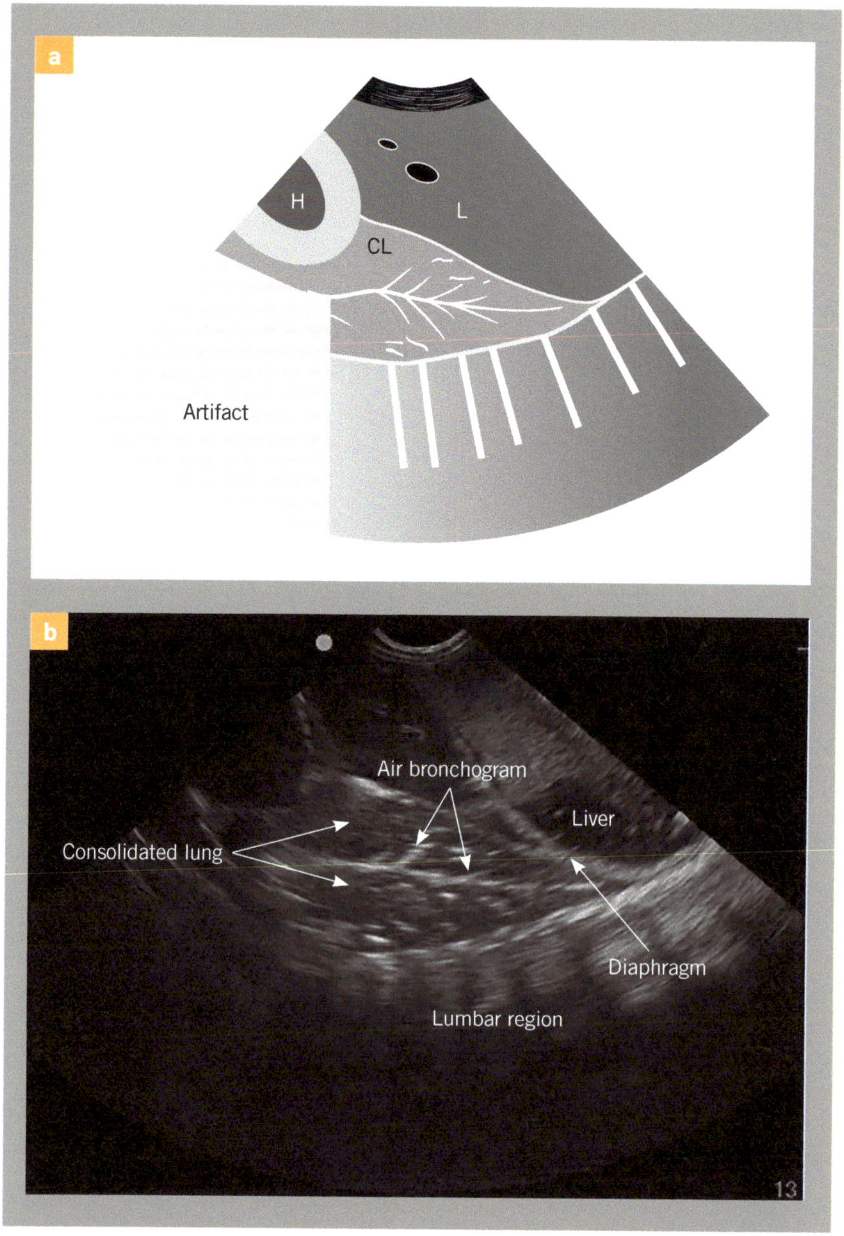

Figure 20. Subxiphoid window schematic and still ultrasound images of full thickness lung consolidation referred to as translobar consolidation. In these images air bronchograms are visible (hyperechoic linear and punctate areas in the still image, white lines in the schematic). An acoustic shadow can be seen (labelled Artifact) arising from trapped air contained within the air bronchogram, which extends to the far field, obscuring structures below it. L; liver, H; Heart, CL; consolidated lung. Image courtesy of Céline Pouzot-Nevoret.

When fluid accumulation in the lungs is severe, the smaller airways may also become fluid-filled, giving rise to fluid bronchograms[9,10]. It is possible to find both fluid and air bronchograms within the same consolidated region of lung or in different regions of the same lung lobe (Fig. 21). Fluid bronchograms can be difficult to differentiate from pulmonary vessels, although some fluid bronchograms may have air visible in addition to fluid, which helps confirm they are fluid bronchograms. Doppler imaging can also be used to differentiate vessels and fluid bronchograms although patient and lung movement make this more challenging in veterinary patients.

If air bronchograms are present are they static or dynamic?

When bronchioles within consolidated lung remain patent, communicating with the large airways, changes in air movement with tidal volume may create visible movement of air within the smaller airways[9,10]. This visible air movement is referred to as a dynamic air bronchogram, and appears similar to the shimmer of lung sliding (Fig. 22; video 7.16). With both partial and translobar consolidations, the movement of air within the airways may still be visible during the respiratory cycle even if lung sliding at the pleural line is absent. In cases, where there is no movement of air within the airways (e.g. resorption atelectasis, lower airway obstruction), a static air bronchogram may be seen. In some instances, an acoustic shadow arises from trapped air contained within an air bronchogram extending through the far field, obscuring consolidated lung tissue below it (Fig. 20; video 7.16).

QR

Video 7.16.
Dynamic air bronchogram (video courtesy Dr. Céline Pouzot-Nevoret, with permission).

Air bronchograms

Air bronchograms are important to identify as they indicate the presence of at least some air within the larger airways in the face of consolidated lung, and can be used to help classify the type of consolidation and possibly the underlying cause.

- Dynamic air bronchograms are most often seen with pneumonia and inflammatory causes of lung consolidation.
- Static air bronchograms are often seen with atelectasis but can also be seen with inflammatory causes of lung consolidation.
- A complete lack of air bronchograms is suggestive of complete atelectasis although severe pneumonia or lobar hemorrhage cannot be excluded. Complete atelectasis is observed during selective intubation.

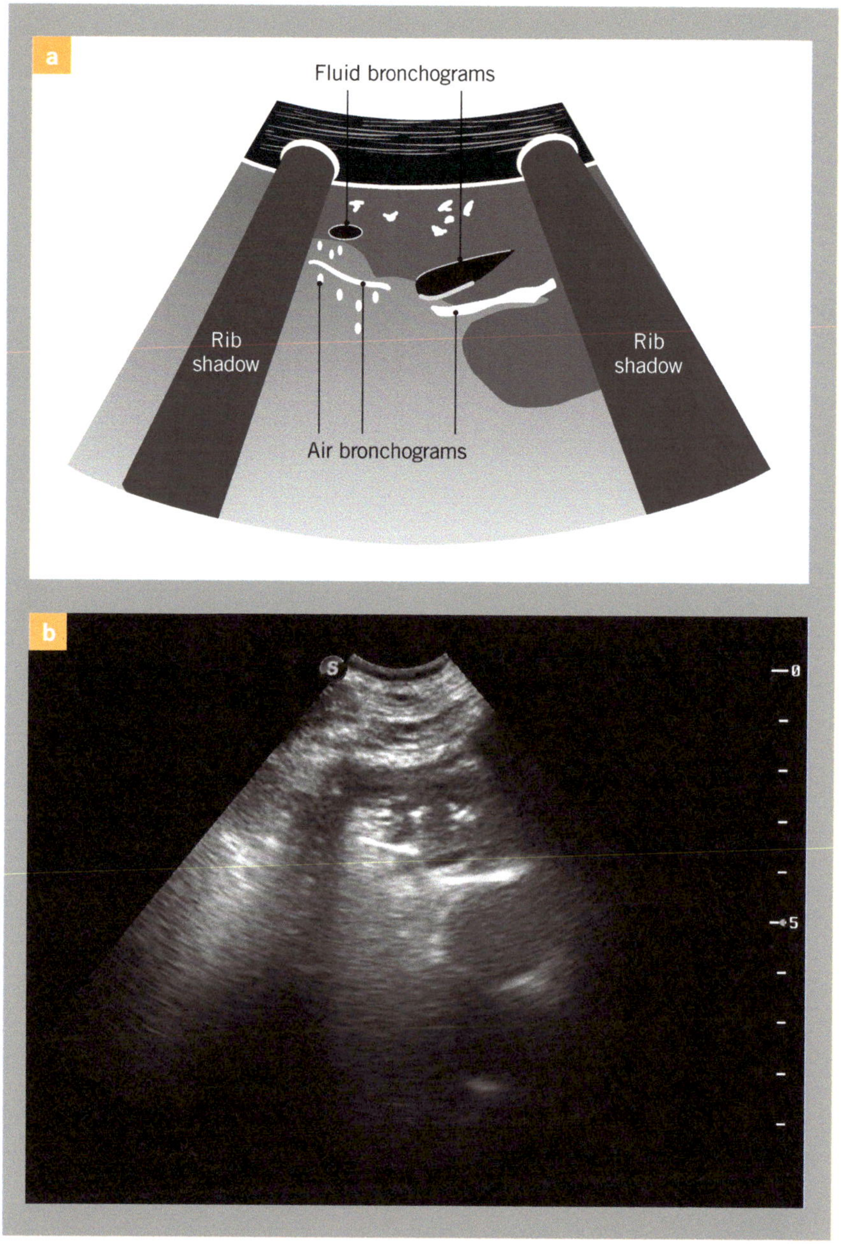

Figure 21. Partial lung lobe consolidation that contains punctate and linear hyperechoic to white regions representing air bronchograms and anechoic round to linear structure, representing fluid bronchograms. Fluid bronchograms can be difficult to differentiate from pulmonary vessels, although some fluid bronchograms may have air visible in addition to fluid, which helps confirm they are fluid bronchograms. Doppler imaging can also be used to differentiate vessels and fluid bronchograms although patient and lung movement make this more challenging in veterinary patients.

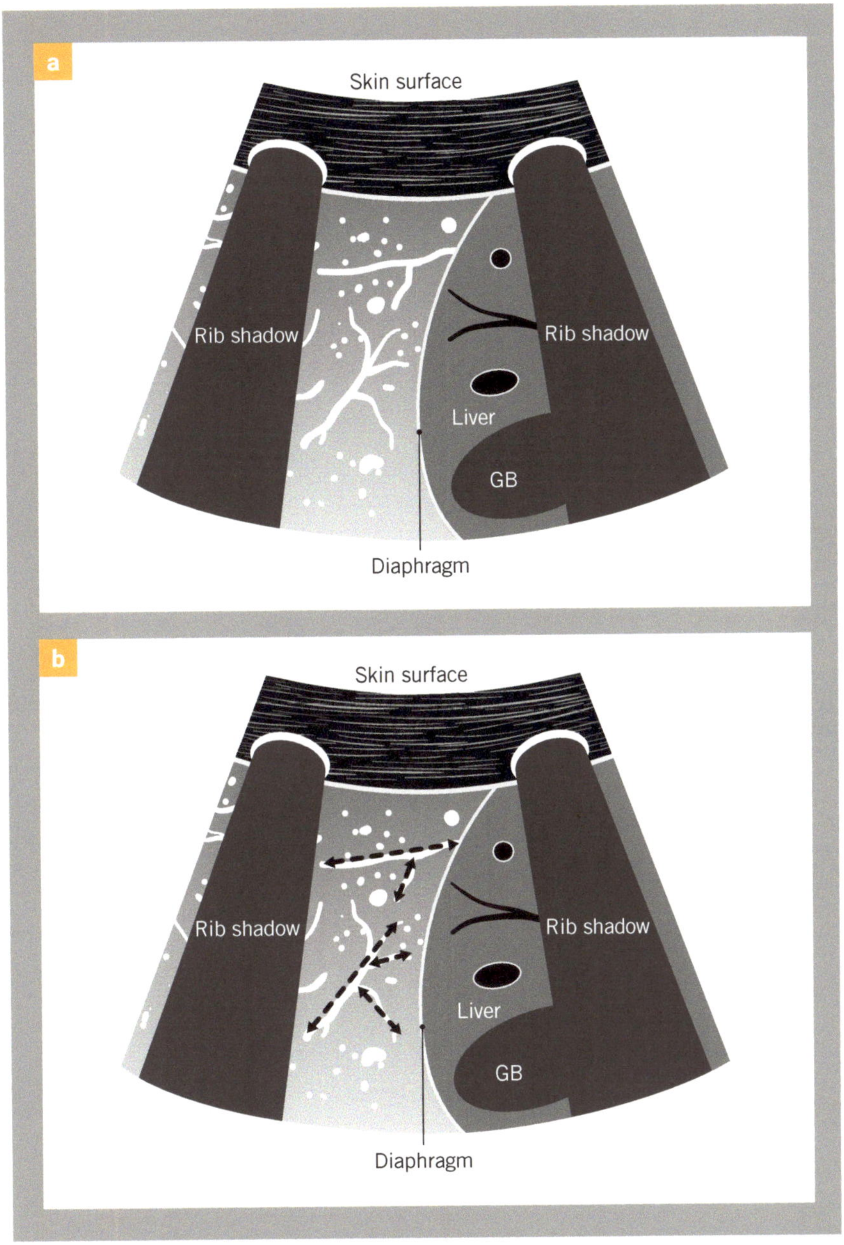

Figure 22. Schematic ultrasound images despicting the difference between static and dynamic air bronchograms. Translobar consolidation is shown with white hyperechoic punctate to linear structures representing air within bronchioles, referred to as air bronchograms. Air bronchograms can be classified as static: no visible air movement within the air bronchogram (a). Air bronchograms can be classified as dynamic: air visible moving within the air bronchogram with respiration, depicted by the black dotted arrow (b). Moving air tends to be visible on inspiration and disappears on expiration. GB; gallbladder.

Is lung volume preserved or decreased?

Although not specific, determining if lung volume is preserved or decreased may help point the clinician towards a diagnosis of atelectasis vs. other causes of lung consolidation[9,10]. When aerated lung tissue is replaced by fluid or cells lung volume tends to be preserved, while lung volume is generally decreased when alveoli become deflated or collapsed secondary to atelectasis (Fig. 23; video 7.17).

Decreased lung volume can be easy to detect on ultrasound when compressed lung is surrounded by pleural effusion; however, it is more difficult to detect with other causes of atelectasis where the lung remains in contact with the thoracic wall (e.g. resorptive and gravitational atelectasis)[9,10]. As the types of atelectasis appear similar on ultrasound, history and other clinical findings are necessary to help determine the likelihood of each.

Although there are several subclassifications of atelectasis, most veterinary patients fall into 1 of 3 general categories:

- **Resorptive (obstructive) atelectasis** as a result of complete airway obstruction. With resorptive atelectasis, the entire lung lobe is often affected creating translobar consolidations as opposed to shred signs.
- **Passive (aka compressive) atelectasis:** as a result of the visceral and parietal pleural being separated (e.g. pleural effusion, pneumothorax, and diaphragmatic hernia, etc). The lung is typically decreased in volume due to the pressure exerted on the lung by pleural space disease.
  - In severe forms of passive atelectasis translobar consolidation is often seen.
  - A mix of increased B lines, shreds and translobar consolidations may be seen with less severe forms of passive atelectasis.

  In case of pneumothorax, the ultrasound beams will be reflected by the air in the pleural space, impeding the visualization of deeper lying atelectatic lung. This implies that the most common cause of compressive atelectasis identified on PLUS will be pleural effusion. The combination of the hypoechoic pleural fluid, decreased lung volume, and a hyperechoic appearance of consolidated lung, results in what has been termed a "jellyfish" sign (Fig. 24; video 7.18).
- **Gravity-dependent atelectasis** which occurs in the most dependent portions of the lungs and may occur secondary to prolonged recumbency and/or general anesthesia.

QR
Video 7.17: Preserved and decreased lung volume with atelectasis.

QR
Video 7.18. "Jellyfish" sign.

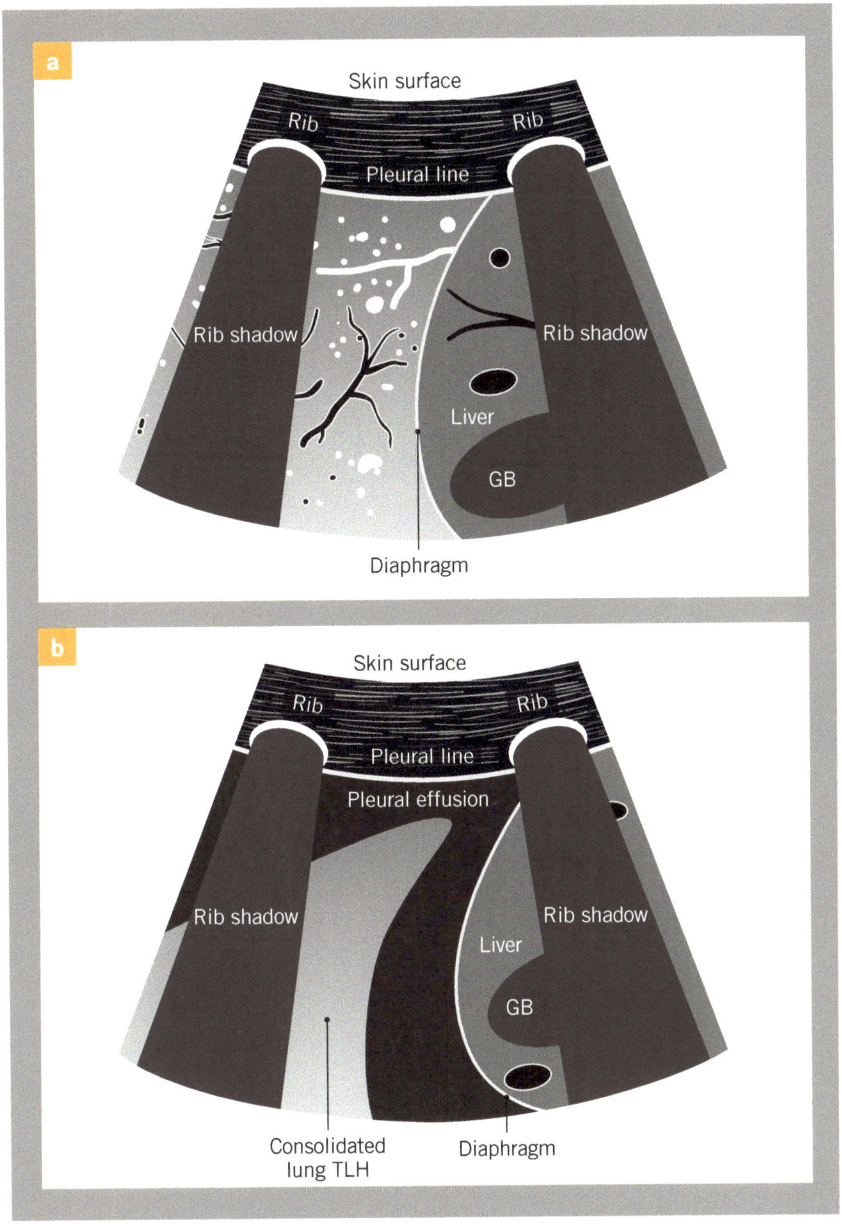

Figure 23. Schematic ultrasound images depicting preserved lung volume (a) and decreased lung volume (b). Although it is not always easy to tell with ultrasound, determining if the lung volume is preserved or not can help determine if the underlying cause is due to atelectasis (lung volume often not preserved) or other causes of lung consolidation (lung volume often preserved). GB; gallbladder, TLH; translobar hepatization.

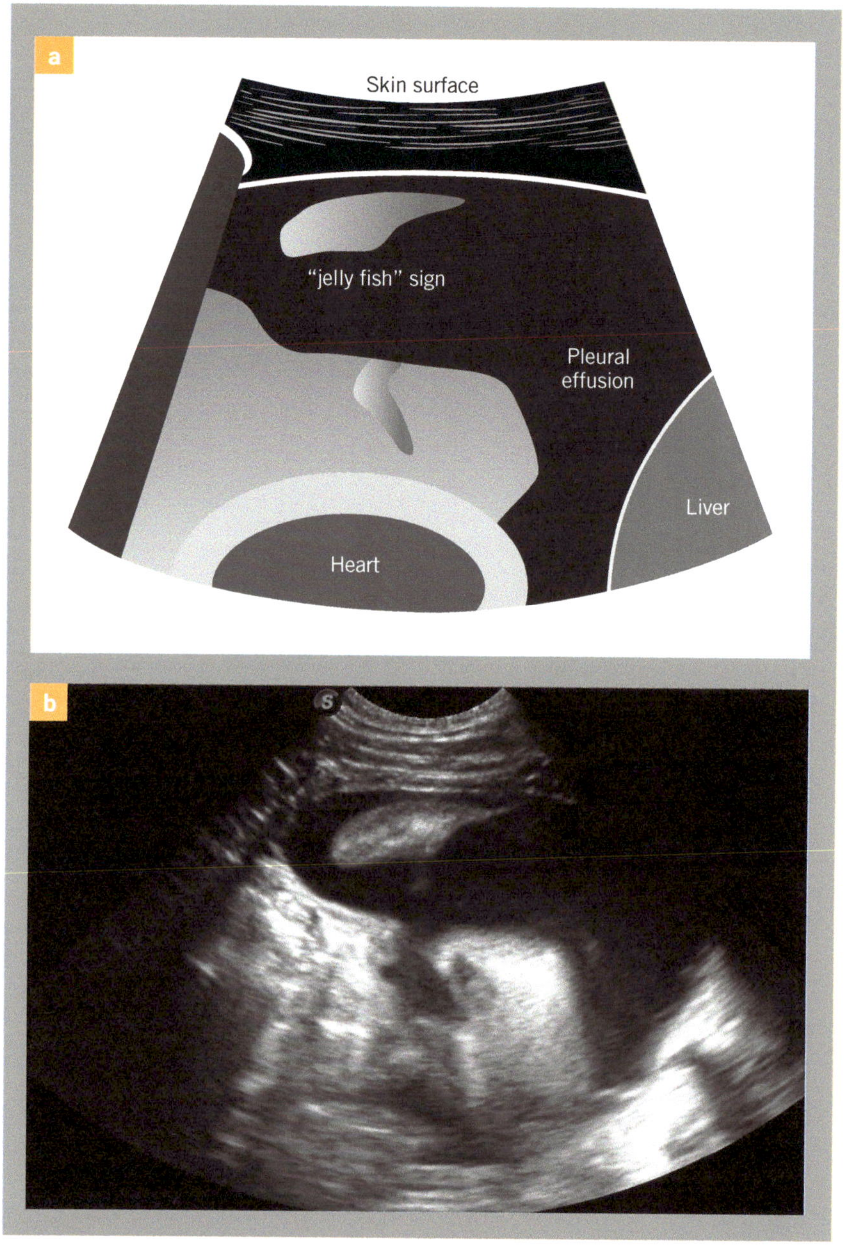

Figure 24. Schematic (a) and still ultrasound images (b) of compressive atelectasis with a small consolidated region of lung visible "floating" in the fluid which is referred to as the "jellyfish" sign.

If air bronchograms are observed with atelectasis, they are typically static (see air bronchograms) due to a lack of air movement within the airways (secondary to low tidal volume or obstructive airway disease)[9].

The presence or absence of a lung pulse in combination with the clinical setting can help identify possible underlying causes of consolidation[8]. The lung pulse is defined by the absence of lung sliding with respiration but the presence of sonographically detectable motion of the lung due to the beating of the heart. The combination of translobar consolidation, absence of lung sliding, and a lung pulse during anesthesia is suggestive of complete atelectasis due to selective intubation[1].

In clinical practice a combination of consolidations is often present in the same patient. For example, a patient with pleural effusion secondary to pulmonary neoplasia may have lung consolidation secondary to passive atelectasis (pleural effusion), but also have lung consolidation due to aerated lung tissue being replaced by neoplastic cells. Therefore, the operator should interpret lung consolidation with caution when there is a loss of lung volume. In other words, consolidation due to neoplasia or other pathology, which tends to carry a worse prognosis, may by masked by the presence of passive atelectasis. Reassessing lung consolidation following therapeutic thoracocentesis is strongly recommended to help differentiate atelectatic consolidation from other causes of consolidation. Furthermore, performing a complete PLUS protocol to establish the entire PLUS profile will also help determine the underlying cause.

Key concepts

- Inflammatory conditions that result in increased extravascular lung water such as contusions, aspiration pneumonia, and acute respiratory distress syndrome are believed to be the most common causes of lung ultrasound consolidation in small animals.
- Left sided congestive heart failure and fluid overload are common causes of increased B lines but uncommon causes of lung consolidations.
- Metastatic neoplasia, fungal disease and abscesses may cause "nodule signs".
- Pulmonary thromboembolism is not well studied but should be suspected when isolated "wedge signs" are detected, particularly with other clinical findings support prothrombotic conditions.

DIAGNOSTIC APPROACH

Lung consolidations can be identified anywhere over the lung surface, and findings may vary within a lung lobe or even within the ultrasound image. The presence or absence of pleural space disease may also help differentiate underlying causes (e.g. pleural effusion and passive atelectasis), hence it is important to scan multiple regions of the lung as well as the pleural space to create the entire PLUS profile. The authors perform a full PLUS exam to decrease the likelihood of missing focal lung consolidations (see Chapter 2). Furthermore, patients with lung consolidation often present with severe respiratory signs; detecting these lesions using PLUS as opposed to other medical imaging modalities decreases patient risk and guides further decision making.

TRANSDUCER ORIENTATION AND SELECTION

A microconvex curvilinear transducer is used by the authors to search for lung consolidation. A lower frequency setting can be used and the depth can be increased to allow most translobar consolidation to be thoroughly assessed. With smaller partial consolidations (e.g. "nodules" and "shred signs"), a linear array transducer may also be used; the larger footprint obtained enables examination of a wider field of the lung surface and higher frequency setting allow greater resolution to assess characteristics contained within consolidations. Similar to identifying other PLUS pathology, the depth is generally set at 2–6 cm, but can be increased if translobar consolidation is encountered. Scanning can be performed with the transducer orientated either perpendicular to or parallel to the ribs. A parallel orientation allows more lung surface to be visualized and may be more sensitive for detection of focal pathology (e.g. nodules and wedge signs). For novice sonographers, perpendicular orientation allows for easier recognition of normal structures via identification of the "bat sign" (See Chapter 3). The authors generally scan with the transducer perpendicular to the ribs when looking for lung consolidations.

PATIENT POSITIONING

Lung consolidations can be identified in any lung field. As lung consolidation does not occur until a lung region has less than 5–10 % air present, most veterinary patients with lung consolidations present with significant respiratory distress. It is advised to scan patients in the position they are most comfortable, which is typically standing or in sternal recumbency (see Chapter 2). In some instances, patients may need to be scanned in lateral recumbency due to concurrent injuries (e.g. spinal fractures). In these patients gravity dependent atelectasis may develop secondary to prolonged lateral recumbency, which may alter the PLUS findings. Ultrasound may need to be repeated after changing the patient position, or following administration of positive pressure ventilation in severely affected patients, which should allow more accurate assessment of PLUS findings.

SONOGRAPHIC TECHNIQUE TO IDENTIFY LUNG CONSOLIDATION

Unlike the diagnosis of pleural effusion and pneumothorax where patient positioning and gravitational effects influence where pathology will accumulate, lung consolidation rarely changes with patient position. However, similar to pleural effusion and pneumothorax, knowing where pathology is most likely to be identified, based on the underlying disease process will increase the sensitivity of finding lung consolidations (e.g. aspiration pneumonia tends to accumulate in the cranial ventral regions).

Furthermore, understanding if consolidations are likely to be focal, lobar or diffuse and mapping the ultrasound patterns to create the PLUS profile will also narrows the differential diagnosis (table 2). To map the lung regions the authors use an "S" shaped scanning protocol, which covers the dorsal third, middle third and ventral third of the thorax, incorporating multiple lung regions within the sonographically defined lung borders (Fig 25; see Chapter 2). In the ventral regions the authors turn the transducer parallel to the ribs, sliding on and off the ventral lung and pleural borders (see Chapter 2).

PITFALLS

As mentioned, lung consolidations can only be detected if the lesions reach the lung surface; deeper isolated pulmonary consolidation that is separated from the lung surface by air will not be visible. Early stages of disease that don't originate at the lung surface may be

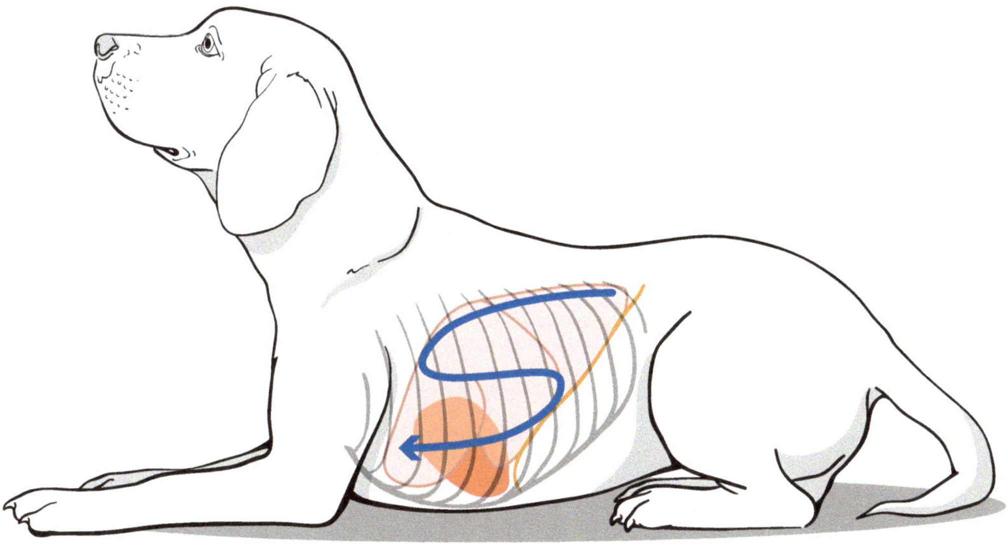

Figure 25. Schematic image depicting the "S" shaped lung pattern the authors use to scan multiple lung regions for pathology. Starting in the caudal dorsal region, a few centimeters below the transition zone from lung to hypaxial/sublumbar muscle and just cranial to the curtain sign, multiple lung regions are assessed in the dorsal third, middle third and ventral third of the thorax following the blue curved arrow. In the ventral regions the transducer is orientated parallel to the ribs as described in Chapter 2 to ensure both the ventral pleural border and ventral lung borders are assessed (not shown in the diagram).

missed; serial examination may detect lesions over time if they progress to involve the lung surface. As only 2/3rd of the lung surface can be scanned, smaller lesions that are hidden below bone (e.g. ribs, scapula) and/or muscle (e.g. sublumbar, shoulder muscles), may go undetected.

Using the PLUS approach limits the likelihood of missing clinically significant lesions.

Extending the forelimb cranially expands the lung area that can be scanned. To avoid a false positive or false negative diagnosis of lung consolidation the operator must be familiar with normal sonographic PLUS borders (see Chapter 2), as well as normal artifacts such as mirror image artifact (Chapter 3). There are several pitfalls that can result in a false positive diagnosis of lung consolidation:

- The mediastinal triangle located at the pericardiodiaphragmatic window can be mistaken for lung consolidation (see Chapter 3).
- With translobar consolidation, because the entire width of the lobe is affected, the soft tissue like lung pattern is easy to mistake for soft tissue organs (e.g. herniated liver, spleen etc.).
- Diaphragmatic and pericardial-peritoneal herniations can often be mistaken for lung consolidations, particularly in the caudoventral regions of the thorax.
- Abdominal structures visible at the curtain sign (transition zone from the lung to the soft tissue structures of abdomen) can be mistaken for consolidated lung (See Chapter 3).
- Mirror image artifact can be mistaken for lung consolidation (See Chapter 3). At the subxiphoid site, the interface between the liver (soft tissue) and the air of healthy lung (or contained in the pleural space in case of a pneumothorax) can create a mirror artifact that resembles lung consolidation. Fanning the transducer to the right of midline until the gallbladder is mirrored on both sides of the diaphragm creates an image artifact that is more easily differentiated from lung consolidation (Fig. 26).

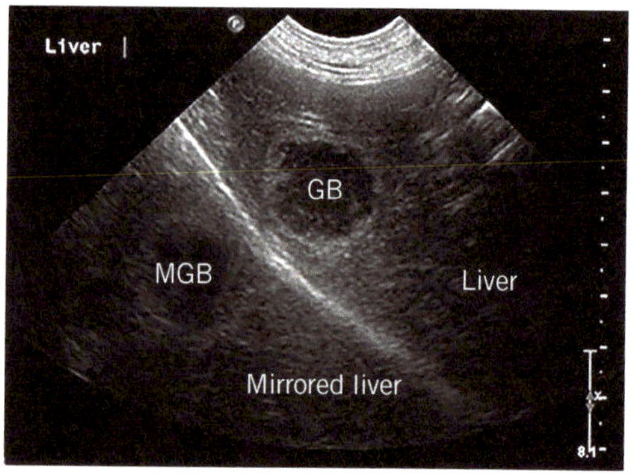

Figure 26. Still ultrasound image of mirror image artifact. The liver is mirrored on the far side of the diaphragm, which can easily be mistaken for consolidated lung tissue. However, if the transducer is fanned to the right of midline while in long axis to the liver, the gallbladder can be identified, which is also mirrored distal to the diaphragm. Detecting the gallbladder helps confirm the sonographic image beyond the diaphragm is mirror image and not lung consolidation. GB; gallbladder, MGB; mirrored gallbladder.

Careful consideration of transducer location, assessing the lung field from different windows (transthoracic as well as from the subxiphoid view), recognizing normal landmarks such as the heart, liver, diaphragm as well as the spleen, and being able to identify the normal sonographic structures of the pericardio-diaphragmatic window are important to decrease the risk of false positives for lung consolidation (see Chapters 2 and 3).

- If pneumothorax is present (See Chapter 4) the lung cannot be assessed for consolidation at that transducer location because the lung is separated from the thoracic wall by a layer of air that prevents the ultrasound beam from reaching the lung surface. Therapeutic thoracocentesis should be performed and PLUS repeated; if lung sliding is visible the lung surface can be assessed for the presence or absence of consolidations.
- If pleural effusion is present, overinterpretation of lung consolidation should be avoided as passive atelectasis can cause consolidation that masks other underlying causes of consolidation (e.g. consolidation caused by fluid or cells replacing aerated tissue). Therapeutic thoracocentesis should be performed and PLUS repeated several minutes later once pleural effusion is no longer present.
- Subcutaneous emphysema inhibits the operators' ability to assess the lung for consolidation as air present in the subcutaneous tissues will prevent the ultrasound beam from reaching the lung surface.
- Lung sliding is unreliable in diagnosing lung consolidation as the pleural line may be attenuated or absent between a region of consolidation and the thoracic wall.

Key concepts

- The identification of hypoechoic tissue, which may contain hyperechoic structures, is indicative of lung consolidation.
- A false positive diagnosis of lung consolidation can occur when:
  - Abdominal organs are mistaken for lung consolidation in the caudal thorax at the level of the curtain sign.
  - Diaphragmatic or pericardial-peritoneal herniations are mistaken for consolidated lung.
  - The normal mediastinal triangle at the pericardio-diaphragmatic window is mistaken for a triangular shaped lung consolidation.
  - Mirror image artifact reflects abdominal organs beyond the diaphragm at the subxiphoid site.
- Performing a complete PLUS exam, identifying sonographic borders of the lung and pleural space, and becoming familiar with the sonographic appearance of normal anatomic structures will decreases the likelihood of both false positive and false negative findings.

PLUS LUNG ULTRASOUND PROFILES

There are three steps to determine the lung ultrasound profile of a patient:

- Answer binary PLUS questions within each ultrasound window.
- Assess regions immediately adjacent to any abnormal lung ultrasound findings.
- Assess PLUS regions over an entire hemithorax, both pleural and lung regions.

The lung ultrasound profile must then be considered with other POCUS findings, history and any additional clinical findings to arrive at the most likely underlying cause.

Within an ultrasound window, binary questions are answered to assess the characteristic lung ultrasound patterns. Although lung ultrasound patterns have not been investigated extensively in veterinary medicine, they are well established in human medicine and should be assessed in small animals.

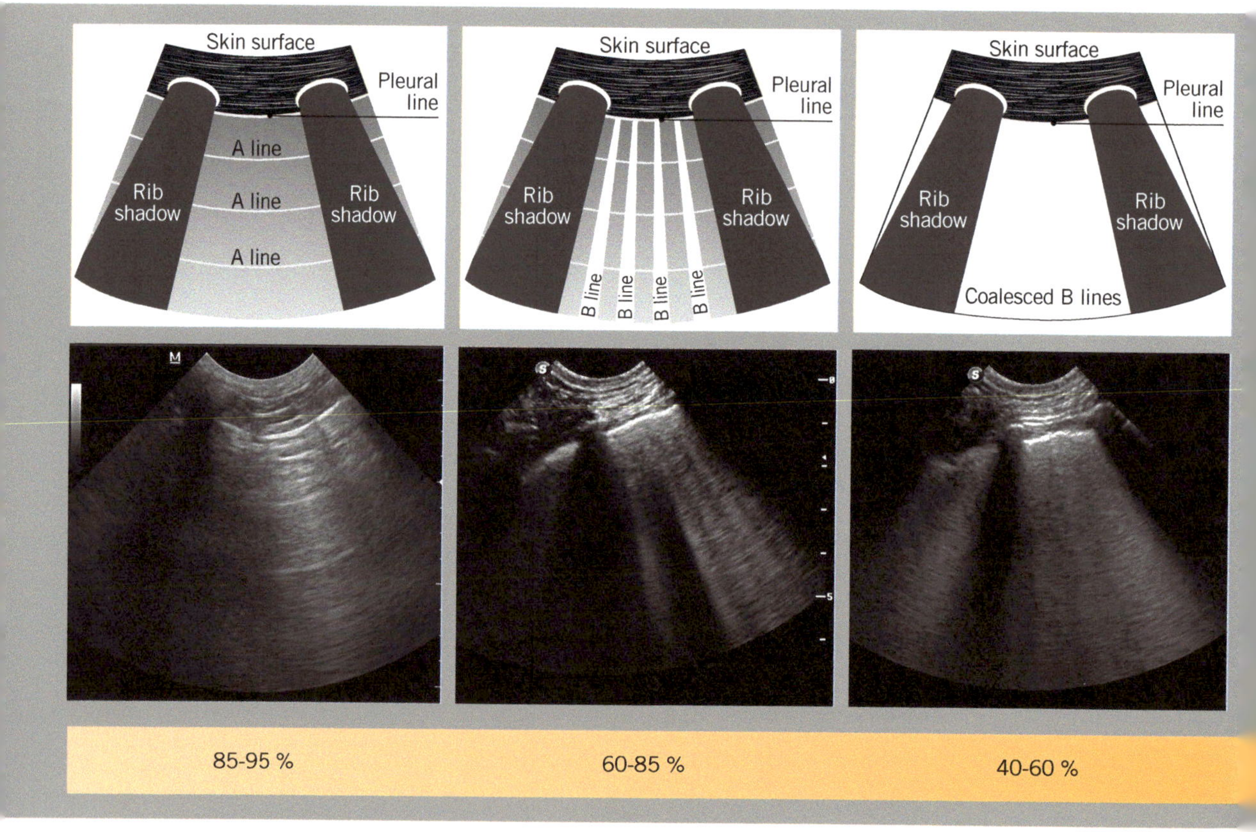

Figure 27. Schematic and still ultrasound images. Different lung ultrasound artifact is detectable when the ratio of aerated to non-aerated lung decreases just below the lung surface. The orange arrow represents the relative percentage of aerated lung, which decreases from the left to right. Far left; healthy air filled lung (85–95 % air). In this setting the lung appears dry and A lines may be visible throughout the far field of the image. In the second image from the left the lung contains less air (say for example 60–85 %), resulting in an increased number of B lines being visible at the lung surface. In the middle image a further decrease in the ratio of aerated to non-aerated lung (say for example 40–60 %) results in B lines being more numerous to the point they begin

Understanding how the appearance of sonographic artifact changes with the progression from healthy lung to consolidated lung helps with understanding the underlying pathology and how to interpret PLUS profiles. Classically, as the ratio of aerated to non-aerated lung below the visceral pleura decreases, a progression from A lines to increased B lines, to coalescent B lines (with or without a thickened pleura/pleural line), to lung consolidation may be seen (Fig. 27).

Although a progression from A lines through B lines to consolidation is often present in patients, consolidation can occur independent of B lines; it is the underlying pathology that dictates the progression and pattern of abnormalities seen, hence the value of assessing PLUS profiles.

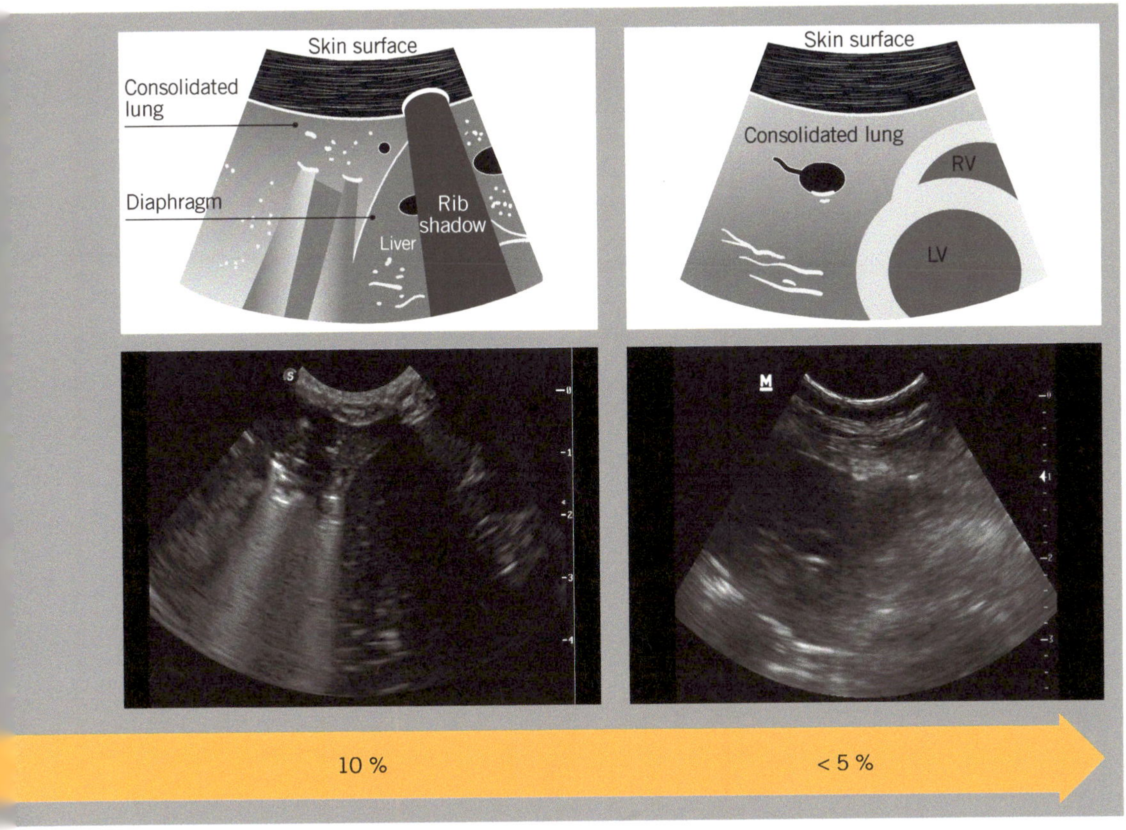

to coalesce. In addition to increased B lines the pleural line may also start to become thickened, irregular and develop a "moth eaten" appearance, which is often considered a precursor to consolidation. When there is less than 5–10 % aerated lung the ultrasound beam is no longer reflected from the lung surface allowing it transverse the lung similar to any soft tissue structure. In the second image from the right lung consolidation is visible, containing air bronchograms. When most of the air is replaced by fluid (≤ 5 % air remaining) fluid bronchograms may become visible in addition to air bronchograms. With resolution of pathology the reverse pattern is often seen from right to left. LV; left ventricular lumen, RV; right ventricular lumen.

In some cases, the cause of respiratory distress can be determined with a high degree of accuracy using PLUS findings alone. For example, pneumonia is often regional, and in case of aspiration pneumonia is located cranioventrally. "Shred signs" and/or translobar consolidation, depending on the extent of the pneumonia, can be identified. The lung tissue immediately adjacent to areas of consolidation often contain increased numbers of B lines (often coalescent), which tend to decrease in severity towards the more caudal and dorsal lung regions. Air bronchograms, often dynamic, and fluid bronchograms, or a combination of the two can often be identified within the consolidated regions. With aspiration pneumonia a lobar sign is often present, as the right middle lung lobe is typically affected in most dogs. The lung volume is generally preserved, and has an echogenicity similar to that of the liver. If necrosis or abscessation develops, the lung lobe will contain well-defined central hypoechoic areas, which may resemble nodules in some cases.

- With lung nodules and thromboembolism isolated partial lung consolidations can be found without the concurrent presence of true B lines.
- Given any combination of lung ultrasound findings can occur in the same patient, within the same hemithorax, or even within the same lung lobe, describing the lung ultrasound signs including thickened irregular pleura, increased numbers of B lines, small subpleural consolidations, "shred signs" and translobar consolidation, as well as any surrounding pleural space pathology is recommended to gather a complete PLUS profile for the patient (Table 2).

SUMMARY

Performing a full PLUS examination increases the chance of identifying focal lung consolidations. Care must be taken to avoid unnecessary patient stress during any POCUS exam, which may dictate the length and starting point of PLUS. By applying the binary question approach to ultrasound identified lung consolidations the operator can rapidly and accurately assess aspects of lung consolidation to further characterize the lesion. Although ultrasound is very sensitive at detecting lung consolidation arising from the lung surface it is not specific with regards to the underlying pathophysiology; atelectasis vs increased fluid and cell content, or a combination thereof. Combining the binary approach with mapping ultrasound findings within and between regions creates the PLUS profile which combined with other POCUS, history and clinical findings refines the diagnosis. The extent to which lung consolidation findings correlate to those described in human medicine remains to be determined.

Table 2. PLUS profiles based on preliminary companion animal data, extrapolation from the human literature, and the clinical experience of the authors.

Pulmonary pathology	PLUS profile findings
Pneumothorax	■ No lung sliding ■ Lung point (hard to find) ■ Abnormal curtain signs (asynchronous/double) ■ A lines visible (parietal pleura reflection)
Pleural effusion	■ No lung sliding ■ Visible separation of the parietal and visceral pleura (may need to extend depth if large pleural effusion is present) ■ ± Consolidation (partial and/or translobar) ■ ± "Jellyfish" sign ■ ± B lines
Pneumonia	■ Shred signs, translobar signs ■ Thickened irregular pleura ■ Subpleural consolidation ■ Unilateral or bilateral B lines ■ Possible small pleural effusion ■ Reduced lung sliding due to consolidations in severe cases ■ Dynamic air bronchograms ■ ± Static air bronchograms ■ ± Fluid bronchograms
Cardiogenic pulmonary edema and fluid overload	■ Widespread and bilateral B lines ■ Coalescing B lines with increasing severity ■ Normal lung sliding ■ Possible bilateral effusion depending on the severity and species (e.g. more common in cats)
Acute respiratory distress syndrome (ARDS)	■ Bilateral or unilateral B lines ■ Normal lung sliding ■ Shred signs, transolobar signs ■ Mixed pattern with spared regions
Feline asthma	■ A lines visible ■ Reduced lung sliding with overinflation ■ ± B lines and consolidation, particularly if right middle lung lobe affected
Pulmonary embolism (PE)	■ Normal lung sliding ■ ± Wedge sign ■ Right ventricular enlargement may be seen with massive/submassive PE
Atelectasis	■ Partial and translobar consolidation ■ B lines often visible ■ ± Static air bronchograms ■ Absence of dynamic bronchograms ■ Reduced lung volume: easy to detect with compressive atelectasis due to pleural effusion

REFERENCES

1. Miller A. Practical approach to lung ultrasound. *BJA Education*, 2016;16(2):39–45.
2. Picano E, Pellikka PA. Ultrasound of extravascular lung water: a new standard for pulmonary congestion. *Eur Heart J*. 2016, 37(27):2097–2104.
3. Lichtenstein DA. Current misconceptions in lung ultrasound: a short guide for experts. *Chest*, 2019, 156(1):21–25.
4. Lichtenstein DA, Mezière GA. Relevance of lung ultrasound in the diagnosis of acute respiratory failure: the BLUE protocol. *Chest*, 2008, 134(1):117–125.
5. Soldati G, Sher S, Testa A. Lung and ultrasound: time to "reflect". *Eur Rev Med Pharmacol Sci*, 2011, 15(2):223–227.
6. Cereda M, Xin Y, Goffi A, et al. Imaging the Injured Lung: Mechanisms of action and clinical use [published correction appears in Anesthesiology. 2019, 131(2):451]. *Anesthesiology*, 2019, 131(3):716–749.
7. Lichtenstein DA, Lascols N, Mezière G, Gepner A. Ultrasound diagnosis of alveolar consolidation in the critically ill. *Intensive Care Med*, 2004, 30(2):276–281.
8. Di Serafino M, Notaro M, Rea G, et al. The lung ultrasound: facts or artifacts? In the era of COVID-19 outbreak. *Radiol Med*, 2020;125(8):738–753.
9. Sperandeo M, Filabozzi P, Varriale A, et al. Role of thoracic ultrasound in the assessment of pleural and pulmonary diseases. *J Ultrasound*. 2008;11(2):39–46.
10. Dietrich CF, Mathis G, Cui XW, et al. Ultrasound of the pleurae and lungs. *Ultrasound Med Biol*, 2015, 41(2):351–365.
11. Ward JL, Lisciandro GR, Ware WA, Miles KG, Viall AK, DeFrancesco TC. Lung ultrasonography findings in dogs with various underlying causes of cough. *J Am Vet Med Assoc*, 2019, 255(5):574–583.
12. Armenise A, Boysen RS, Rudloff E, et al. Veterinary-focused assessment with sonography for trauma-airway, breathing, circulation, disability and exposure: a prospective observational study in 64 canine trauma patients. *J Small Anim Pract*, 2019, 60(3):173–182.
13. Rodrigues N, Giraud L, Billen F, et al. Comparison of thoracic point of care ultrasound and radiographic findings as well as clinical evolution and C Reactive Protein concentrations in dogs treated for aspiration pneumonia. *Ultrasound J*, 2020,12(Suppl 1): 45.
14. Reissig A, Kroegel C. Transthoracic ultrasound of lung and pleura in the diagnosis of pulmonary embolism: a novel non-invasive bedside approach. *Respiration*, 2003, 70(5):441–452.
15. Hatabu H, Uematsu H, Nguyen B, et al. CT and MR in pulmonary embolism: A changing role for nuclear medicine in diagnostic strategy. *Semin Nucl Med*, 2002, 32(3):183–192.